A book from The Fasted Way Method

FAST TILL DINNER ONCE PER WEEK

The *rule* Breaker's Guide To *weightloss*

A 120-DAY FASTING GUIDE;
Learn the method, lose the weight.

Elisabeth Gabelmann

the rule breaker's guide to weight loss.

Your 120-Day Fasting Schedule

elisabeth gabelmann

fasted publiahing co.

contents

dedication

To my father-in-law, Bill.
Encouragement can come from the most unlikely places. It went through a casual conversation with my father-in-law with an "out of the blue" comment.
"Hey," he said. "I've been fasting once a week." There must have been some surprise on my face. "You have?" I responded. "Yeah," Bill continued, "I like what you said about supplements, that we put too much focus on them and not enough on the other things we're supposed to be doing." I was still surprised. "I'm noticing a difference when I fast," he shared. "Bill, that's amazing." I gushed. He then began encouraging me as he knew I was working towards my final goal, which started my entire weight loss journey in January 2023.
"How close are you to your goal?" He asked. "Just seven pounds. I'm so close." I responded. "Well, keep after it. I'm cheering for you." Bill said.
My father-in-law has brought so much value into the world because he loves his family and the company he built. What struck me was that I had something of substance that was

bringing a natural solution to his problem. I don't know if there is a more tremendous honor than contributing to others who work to improve the world.
This book is a result of that conversation.
Bill, thank you!

preface

I am not a medical professional, and this book is not advice. I have no licenses in psychology, psychiatry, nutrition, or exercise. What you will read in this book is solely my opinion.

I went to college to study journalism and have most of my writing experience investigating news story topics. The majority of my life has been spent in sales, with the most extended stint being in two large direct sales companies, where I experienced more success than most. I would say the fourteen years I was actively selling supplements, partnered with becoming a mother, and the biological changes I was unprepared for are two of the most significant contributors to this book.

I was the very picture of a direct seller, I took the products and regurgitated the sales points of each product. After the birth of my second child, I started asking more questions as the product alone, inconsistent workout plans, and living by the 80/20 rule were not giving me the same weight loss results as before. As I ventured out to find answers outside the company I was representing, I began to see the pieces I was missing. I had one driving thought: 'We cannot continue to tell customers to buy more products or a new product line to answer their weight loss problems. There has to be more to the story.'

I love and value supplements and still receive residual payments from products I've recommended. However, I realized that getting the results I wanted would require me to remove supplements as the star of the show and recast them in the supporting, supplemental role they were intended for all along. The contents of this book are the 'more' to the story I hoped I'd find.

Lastly, I can almost guarantee you will find typos. As a part-time, self-publishing author with a visual disability and a full-time mom, perfection is not the goal of this book. While there may be grammatical errors, they should not impede your ability to learn and apply the method to see the weight loss results you know you are capable of. Typos be damned. Perfection is an expensive, mythical unicorn that does not exist. I hope you learn to love the flaws in you as you find them in these pages too.

**You'll find blank pages scattered throughout this book. Use them to write your thoughts or high points you want to remember or go back to and research on your own. The companion study guide has a discount code on the resources page.

resources & free downloads

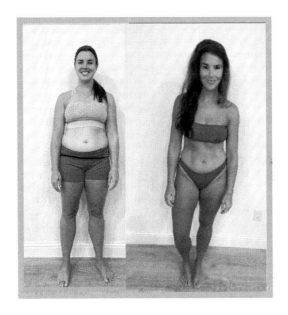

As a valued reader, your purchase of this book entitles you to an exclusive selection of digital downloads. These resources, designed as companions, will enrich your learning journey and provide unique insights.

To get your free and discounted downloads, go to:
www.thefastedway.com

After you type in the corresponding discount code and checkout, these ebooks and guides will automatically be emailed to your inbox. Click on the product you want to download and enter the discount codes below on the checkout page to apply your discount.

- **120-Day Fasting Schedule & checklists** (Code: FREE120)
- **Power Protein Plan $9.99 / discount $2.99** (Code: PROTEINPLAN)
- **Rule Breaker's Study Guide $12.99 /discount $7.99** (Code: STUDY120)
- **Fast On Track Consult - 60 minutes $697 / discount $397** (Code: CONSULT120)
- **This Ain't Your Mama's Fast Mini Course | On-demand-video course $37 / discount $17.97** (Code: MINI120)
- **DIY Weightloss Starter Course | On-Demand-video course $297 / discount $127** (Code: STARTER120)

foreword

The Rule Breakers: Your Invitation to Bend or Break The Weight Loss Rules.

The night stilled the sounds of cannons and gunfire brought with the light of the day. Tensions of religious insistence still hung in the air over the land of what is now modern-day Ukraine, quietly anticipating the first signs of day and the resurgence of war. If you were to listen, there would be no differentiating sound between the groans of dying Russian men and Western Europeans. In this place, where darkness hovered over blood-soaked dirt, pain was the sound of humanity; needs were the same, and death held no discrimination of creed or color.

She lit her lamp as she did every night to walk among them, the men she cared for, the ones she could restore to life, and those she could only administer comfort before death took their hand. They called her "The Lady with the Lamp" as she walked row after row through British Army hospital beds during the Crimean War. What would drive a British woman born to a wealthy, aristocratic family with every privilege at her disposal and given an elite education to abandon modern comfort in exchange for this place?

Perhaps she identified more with the battlefield than drawing rooms and opera houses.

If you know her story, Florence Nightingale was the definition of a rebel. A term that seems to be more associated with recklessness and may conjure up images in your mind of James Dean standing next to his name in red letters for 'A Rebel Without A Cause.' If you remember her story, Nightingale walked the fine line between knowing which rules to bend and which to break. This tendency to bend or break the rules must have run in her family because a young Florence was given an education in math, philosophy, and language, which was rare for female children of the day. It didn't stop there, though. Nightingale continued to break the rule of the day, abandoning societal expectations for women of her class to marry; she said she felt "a call to serve others" and was drawn to the medical field.

If you're at all familiar with the story, you know her path led Florence Nightingale to establish modern nursing, considered to be lowly, unskilled, and unnecessary. But when the death tolls in the Army hospitals were on the rise due to patients laying in their own filth, she was called on by the British government to use the skills she'd fought to acquire in the face of the societal rules her own government upheld. As Nightingale applied her logistical, organizational, and medical skills fueled with compassion her methods decreased the death toll from 42% to 2% in six months.

The Lady with the Lamp was undoubtedly a rule breaker.

It feels like a leap, doesn't it, connecting the ground-breaking stand of an iconic female figure to your modern-day plight to lose ten pounds? When I started this journey, I felt the same. I wanted a 'Nobel quest' to apply my love of writing. In my early journalism days, I wanted to be a wartime journalist. That felt like a worthy cause to devote my life to. Last year when I connected the pillars that would become 'The Fasted Way Method', I remember feeling disappointed and asking this internal question, "Couldn't my path have led towards something more dignified than weight loss?"

After a year of applying this method to my life and walking alongside women I've been able to coach, I can tell you there is a hidden worth in this work that has surprised me. What repulses me, and probably you, about the weight loss industry is the over-glorification of aesthetics and shiny products that are the same price as a hospital stay with your first baby, but bring little results for the long-term.

It honestly feels lowly and gross.

From my perspective, weight loss feels like a marketing playground where women who are desperate to see change in their bodies fall prey to celebrity endorsements and well-made websites.

A few months ago, I was interviewing a friend for another book I am writing and shared my sentiment with her. Jess is a 52-year-old north-easterner who has overcome incredible odds with menopause and is known for her straightforward nature and her 'tell it like it is' narration of her life. Her compassion came through the screen when I shared my disappointment as she responded, "But look at what you're creating? Look what you're doing for women?" It made a profound impact.

Maybe you feel the same way. You aren't taking care of dying soldiers on a battlefield; you are wiping little hineys (that's a southern term of endearment for butts.) You aren't applying ground-breaking science you are doing five loads of laundry. Maybe you'd love to volunteer more, start that business plan tucked away in your office drawer, or attend school board meetings. But the weight you need to lose to feel comfortable in your skin claws at the back of your mind like a squatter in your thoughts that won't vacate to make way for more 'noble enterprises.'

What if creating daily habits that infiltrate your home and create a culture of health was the noble cause, though?

Millennial women are the most health-conscious generation, according to the data, but we are the sickest. Our children suffer from diseases that some medical professionals hadn't even heard of twenty years ago. Perhaps fighting for our health is the best thing we can do.

Women in modern-day America have everything at their fingertips to achieve the most health in the scope of human history. We have resources, we have modern conveniences, but 56% of us are struggling with obesity. It affects everything.

Perhaps you aren't the Florence Nightingale, or Barbara O'Neil of your time, but what if you're raising her? What if she is living in your house right now, and her little eyes are watching and storing the decisions you make for your health? What could be nobler than that: shaping the next generation of women?

This book invites you to think differently about yourself, the mind-body connection, and how you see your body. I won't tell you which weight loss rules to bend or break. You can read the information, ideas, and theories that make up The Fasted Way Method but decide for yourself. That will be the first rule many of you break: deciding for yourself. It's countercultural in 2024 to apply critical thinking skills and problem-solving to your life. The familiar road looks like consuming the marketing messages being fed to us from every angle. Yet, 56% of us are struggling with obesity.

I love having a diverse group of female friends. However,

the most common thread is how often the signs they see about their bodies are dismissed by health professionals. This isn't specific to a particular age group or health issue. If I was struggling with the idea of 'weight loss being noble enough' to be worth my energy, it stopped being a question in my mind when I heard a friend say she was struggling with suicidal thoughts because her health was declining so rapidly. She was being dismissed by every doctor she went to.

As you read 'The Rule Breaker's Guide To Weightloss,' I ask you to lead with curiosity about yourself and an open mind, thinking that maybe there is more to your story than you've been telling yourself.

To bend of break the rules will be entirely up to you.

introduction

Meet Stella.

The table was set. Stella, a 36-year-old mom of three, put the easy meal of chicken nuggets, fries from the air fryer, and last night's pizza on the table with a roll of paper towels in the center for the inevitable spill.

"Dinner is ready!" She sang out. Her voice echoed off the high ceilings of her home, reverberating up the staircase where Avery, Judah, and Simon had lost themselves in the fort building. She hoped to hear feet quickly pointing to her call, but that wasn't the outcome.

"I know they can hear me." She thought.

A second questioning thought quickly followed it, "Can they hear me?"

"Do I go up? Do I call them again?" She asked herself. Meanwhile, the leftover pizza was getting even more "left-over-y," and the clock was ticking. It was time for her to get dressed.

Kristen had asked her to come for a girl's dinner, and in desperate need of that estrogen aura that only comes from other females laughing and eating together, Stella said, "I can't wait." A gloomy thought quickly followed it, and it came out as a question.

Stella asked the question one woman asked another woman after she had been invited out: "What are we wearing? Are we coming as is? Or getting cute?"

Kristen answered, "You can wear whatever you love; I will dress up." What do you suppose Stella immediately decided?

"Crap! Now I must wash my hair and put something on besides my tired mom's uniform." Quick calculations started in her head. How long has it been since I've washed my hair? Could I get away with dry shampoo? Nope. I can smell my head. I am washing. Of course, she didn't say that out loud. "Those are inside thoughts!" Stella always says this to her three offspring when they yell something out of their mouths, and she wishes they hadn't.

Like a winding staircase cascading down the spiral of her mind, her thoughts were quickly hijacked by memories of a different time in her life when "getting dressed" was enjoyable, not dreadful, when 10:00 am pilates and bottomless mimosas at brunch weren't a contradiction because you re-drank all the calories you just burned off in your cute matching set you'd just bought from Lululemon.

She deep sighed. That was three babies and less stress-ago.

"It's not the kids." She would tell her husband, Cal, when he found her deep breathing in their closet. The closet was her soundproof escape place when nervous system overload meant to "get out now" or "stay and face rage mom" were her only two options. The overwhelming thought came from her attempts to find something to wear.

"They're just kids. They do kid stuff. Expecting them to

do or be anything else makes me more frustrated." She would explain.

"It's me. I'm the problem. Why can't my clothes just fit?"

After twelve years of marriage, Cal, a millennial dad who worked a hybrid job for a corporate firm, had figured out that these were not the moments for phrases like "Didn't you just buy something new last summer?" There was one sentence he kept in his pocket that was fail-proof, and he immediately deployed it:

"How can I help?" He asked in an empathetic tone.

Stella quickly looked up at him and smiled, remembering other "fat moments" in their closet when nothing seemed to fit, the clock was ticking, all her friends were going to "look cute," and her well-meaning husband said, "But you have a closet full of clothes." Her smile said, 'Thank you for not trying to fix me.'

Stella responded to his question, "Can I have a hug? And will you get the three monkeys to eat their dinner so I can get dressed in peace?"

The hug always seemed to calm her nervous system, something Stella had been learning more about in attempts to lose the 12-year-old baby weight and be less of a raging mom.

Now, what to wear? "God! I hate this! Can't we just all wear sweats?" She pulled out her classic black, go-to maxi dress that hid the parts of her body she hated the most. She'd spent too much time despairing over how much she hated her body and all the clothes in her closet, so dry shampoo would have to mask her smelly scalp smell. Of course, personal hygiene and showers seem to be things that get put on the back burner more and more these days.

With one glance in the mirror and another deep sigh, she quietly spoke to her reflection, "Stella, where are you?"

With that, she was off to a fun girls' dinner where she would eat a grilled chicken salad when she ordered the ravioli with lobster bisque. She would let herself eat half of a roll because "carbs make you fat! Don't you know that?" She would most assuredly skip dessert because she didn't need those extra calories, and refusing when the server asked made her feel better, as if she was giving all her fat cells an eviction notice that she was stronger after all.

At dinner, the girlfriends swap the latest information they've learned about losing weight fast and discuss plans to 'get in shape,' though all express that they have no idea where to start.

On the way home, Stella stops at 7 11, not to fill up on gas but to grab the ice cream she wished she would've just let herself have at dinner, 'but at least I can go home and put my comfy pants on. Should I get Cal some?"

Stella wants a simple way to care for her body without spending hours in the gym, sacrificing all the food she loves, spending thousands of dollars on supplement programs, and virtually hating her life.

She needs The Fasted Way Method, a compassionate approach to weight loss and health that breaks everything down into bite-size pieces while delivering excellent, lasting results. Are you ready to learn how?

"Don't Remind Me."

I can hear your thoughts crossing sound barriers right now, saying, "I thought this was a book about how to lose weight while fasting, not a novel. I don't want to read this. I live Stella's life every day."

It is. You will get all the tools you need to make fasting a part of your life. But you've read info-only books before, right? Or have you taken a class or hired a coach? Why will this book be any different?

The method puts this book in a category of its own. Equally as important is the approach. The fasting process is only as effective as the approach of self-compassion to guide you through your journey. This book is a guide to getting through your first 120 days of fasting for weight loss. You could read basic info, follow a guide, never connect to your inner world and the demands you have on your daily life, and fail one more thing in an attempt to 'lose that weight.' You only accomplished deepening your belief that 'nothing works for me.' How about we try something different?

Which part of Stella's evening and attempts to get dressed stuck out to you? Don't rush. Take a moment and connect. Please write it down.

Now that you have connected to that moment, why did you relate to that part?

If you've answered those two questions, congrats! You just started The Fasted Way Method.

we start with compassion

How To Use This Book

'Stella' is a fictional compilation of many women who know the crazy ride of 'once upon a time, when guilt wasn't sewn into the fabric of my clothes.' When the jeans seemed to fit, and donuts didn't represent bloating or a five-pound weight gain.

Thankfully, Stella's great friend Kristen doesn't just invite her to girl's dinner, but also buys her and Stella a copy of "The Rule Breaker's Guide To Weight Loss " and asks, "Can we do it together?"

You, Kristen, and Stella will find a compassionate approach to weight loss written in these pages, not an 'all or nothing' doomsday plan. The end of that doomsday story promises you will fail at the first sight of a Nothing Bundt Cake.

"Rule Breakers" is a comprehensive plan to help clarify weight loss confusion while preventing burnout and gives you a solution to the problems you don't know you have.

THE SECTIONS: Where the magic happens.

Section One: What is The Fasted Way Method, and why does it work? As you read this book, you enter a different world where industry terms are explained and new ideas are fertilized. Spoiler: the method works because it teaches you to partner a time-condensed calorie deficit with the power of protein and walking while simultaneously telling women they can keep their Oreos; the only thing you're losing is weight with The Fasted Way Method.

Section Tw0: *"Keep It Basic" You're 8-HR Fast.* This section is written with the go-getters in mind who will want to start the process while reading this book. You will get a sample schedule to follow and see ideas for what to do before, during, and after your fast. The most asked questions are also covered in this section.

Section Three: *"The Internal Lens & The Science Of Compassion."* We will give 1980 their weight loss mentality back, ditch endless Richard Simmons cardio, and treat ourselves compassionately as we learn to set goals. "Go hard, or go home." "I have to be all in to start. " "I fell off the wagon/ track and need to get started again." It won't be phrases you think or say anymore.

Honey-frend-booboo-child (make sure you say that in a southern accent) while you are fixing a wagon wheel and trying to figure out how to get back "on" your 1896 wagon, there is a 'Tesla' with the keys in the ignition waiting for you to jump in for the ride of your life.

"The Wagon" is the traditional approach to weight loss that hasn't worked for you; otherwise, you wouldn't be reading this book looking for something new. "The weight loss wagon" has the word "NO" written on it in big red letters, and underneath those crimson letters are all the foods not allowed on the wagon.

I want you to imagine I just handed you a box of matches. The flame just illuminated, and when you throw it at "the wagon," you say goodbye to everything that "hasn't worked for you in the past." It was set up to fail from the beginning because it is rigid, unforgiving, and never gives room for cake or the demands you have on your daily life. You don't want to live that way anymore.

"The Tesla" is extended fasting fueled by protein and self-compassion for the demands of your everyday life.

Compassionate goal-setting is necessary if you successfully follow the 120-day fasting schedule in this book.

The Science. *T*he Fasted Way Method is built on unchanging scientific facts. Those principles are divided into two parts: the science of living and The Science of weight loss.

The method stems from the fact that you have to eat, drink water, and move your body to live. You must prioritize those three physical essentials while incorporating a calorie deficit and prioritizing protein to lose weight.

Sounds so simple. Simple, yes. Easy? No! The Fasted Way is a delicate recipe of self-compassion, grit, and endurance. None of those attributes are gained quickly but can be attained over time while you see results on the scale in your first 30 days.

How Does It Work?

Covering the five fundamental pillars inside The Fasted Way Method, you'll learn precisely what you need to do to see the results that have constantly alluded to you in the past. Protein, Movement, Water, Supplements, and Autophagy Fasting are all explained and laid out in a comprehensive plan for you to follow for 120 days.

Section Four: *"You've Got The Power: Power Protein, Power Walks, & Wonder In The Water."* Understanding the principles laid out in this section will be crucial to your success. The power of protein sets this method apart from anything else you've read or the weight loss approach you've employed. Knowing how to use protein will ensure your success or failure. Simultaneously, we need to talk about exercise, except we make a 'word exchange' and replace 'exercise' with 'movement.' Because of the hostile and intimidating nature the word exercise can evoke in your thoughts, using the word 'movement' opens up the idea of what can help your body move for overall health. Even better, my method uses walking as the primary means for movement and weight loss. Because walking can be done at any time and location, you are increasing the likelihood of your success by committing to walking. Reading this section, will show you how.

Section Five: *120 DAYS Let's Map Your Plan.*

It takes 21 days to create a new habit. Part of what you're going to learn will be new habits. Your first 30 days implementing this new system will be focused on adjusting. This is new, and nothing new is done perfectly in the beginning. The best part, though, is you can still jump-start results in your first 30 days because an 8-hour fast is just that powerful.

Amanda lost 8 pounds in her first seven days.

Sandra lost three pounds on her first 8-hour fast and 10 pounds on her first thirty days.

Even as you fumble through learning something new, scientific principles don't change, which is why Amanda and Danielle saw results so quickly. To stay focused, you'll need the other four pillars for the marathon race, resulting in a life of beautiful results.

Section Six, "The Final Countdown," covers the last of my tips and tricks for success using The Fasted Way Method. There's also a short chapter on how to use this method with the men in your life.

my isn't broken,

body

it just needs the
right tools to
succeed!

Elisabeth Gabelmann

section
one

THE FASTED WAY METHOD

one

. . .

What Is The Fasted Way Method?

The Fasted Way Method is a combination of two things. First, scientific facts must be embraced to get results from your body. Second are ideas or theories like "Weight loss shouldn't be this hard" that address the emotional impact of the journey. The Fasted Way Method marries body and mind together. You will not find a harsh list of demands for your body or strict statements that ignore your emotional and mental health. If you believe weight loss should be simple, there is only one path forward - find a more straightforward way to get the results you're looking for. You will find what you're looking for if they are thoroughly resolved. The result of that thought is the Fasted Way method, which combines science with compassionate ideas that get accurate results for women amid their busy lives. You'll find a combination of daily actions and core beliefs with deep thought about how women live daily. While this book is not meant to be therapeutic in any way, there will be ideas you'll read that may point you in a direction to have a deeper conversation with a trusted therapist.

. . .

LET'S explore and establish some core beliefs that set this method apart from anything you've tried before. First, your weight is not an indicator, in any way, of your value as a person. Regardless of the number on the label sewn into the back of your jeans, it's not a measure of your moral goodness or "badness." While the tag may measure the size of your waist, and yes, it's okay to want that number to be different, "size 16" cannot be used to calculate the value of your soul. You are not morally good if the number is smaller or morally wrong if the number is more significant.

IN HER BOOK "How To Keep House While Drowning," author KC Davis touches on moral neutrality with care tasks in your home.

"When you view care tasks as 'moral,' the motivation for completing them is often shameful. You don't feel like a failure when everything is in its place. When it's messy or untidy, you do."

As I read her book, I noticed much overlap with the journey of bodily health.

Digging into this broad topic of weight loss, I have encountered some of the most heartbreaking statements escaping the lips of women sharing their stories with me.

"I promise, I don't just sit around and eat all day," a friend told me. She was struggling with health issues related to an overwhelming amount of weight on her body that was taking an extreme toll on her overall health.

My heart broke. I didn't think overeating was the result of her body's weight. What it felt like she was saying to me underneath that statement was, "I'm not lazy."

Davis writes a powerful statement in her book that I must

share before we move on. I hope you will hold it closely as you go through this process.

"I do not think laziness exists. Do you know what does exist? Executive dysfunction, procrastination, feeling over-whelmed, perfectionism, chronic fatigue, depression, lack of skills, lack of support, trauma, and differing priorities."

CORE THOUGHT: **Your plate must always be more precise when adopting new health habits. There will always be non-negotiable "broccoli" on your plate of life. What can you say 'Yes' to today that will move you forward?**

I am not a nutritionist or a trainer; I have no certifications or degrees that would qualify me by most standards on this topic. What I have to offer you as credibility are my results and those of women who've trusted me to walk with them.

JEN IS a 38-year-old millennial mom with one hundred pounds to lose from her 5-foot-4-inch frame. She is strong and vibrant. She is an incredible professional singer and performer. She also sells real estate and is learning to create online courses. Jen is tired, but she is driven.

As our FaceTime call starts, I feel the energy coming through my screen. Jen and her mom, Karla, are excited, with the energy you hope for when helping someone jump-start healthy habits. As I start to share, I can tell they're both waiting on me for something. Finally, Jen blurts out, "Ok, but can you tell us what we need to stay away from? Like a list?"

I sighed deeply, smiling, and said, "We'll focus on what we will do. Not what we aren't going to do." It felt like Jen and Karla held their breath, waiting for me to say, "Just kidding! Go empty your pantry and put all the Oreos in the trash." But I didn't.

CORE THOUGHT: I don't believe in "cheat days," "cheat food," "good food," or "bad food." It's all food. How we use it and the results we get from those foods are up to us. Food is morally neutral.

Jen started with one 8-hour fast per week, one hundred grams of protein, ninety ounces of water, and seven thousand steps throughout her day. She didn't incorporate any supplement program, and I never gave her a list of "don't eat food." We loaded every conversation with compassion for the demands of her life.

Her first fast didn't see the results, and neither of us thought she would. So, we adjusted and used the "Fast On Track Progress Tracker" to see where the gaps were.

One week of tracking and another FaceTime later, the tracker painted the picture I thought it would. Jen struggled to adjust to her protein intake and get all her daily steps in. We slowed down and talked through it. During that phone call, she said, "I think I could do two 24-hour fasts this week." I responded, "Sure, I can get on board with that on one condition," I paused, waiting to complete the sentence.

"If you get to dinner and you're going to lose it on one of your kids because you're hungry, call it quits and eat." She agreed, and I made a mental note to check in with her the next day.

The idea that most of us have when it comes to fasting, working out, eliminating food from our lives, or incorporating a supplement program is that if we do "more" of that thing, we'll get results. We run further and push ourselves harder until our bodies demand nurturing and care. Mentally, "going hard" makes us feel better, but we lack understanding of what is happening in our bodies. It takes so much mental fortitude to get up and be "all in" that even if you have the cognitive energy to start, you won't be able to do it again. Instead, you burn out and make a beeline for the pantry. Your husband finds you sitting on the floor with the peanut butter jar and a spoon.

IF YOU HAVE STRUGGLED with weight gain for the majority of your life, are over the age of thirty-five, or have birthed children, your body is going to require more from you to be able to respond by letting go of the weight. This isn't just true for some people. It is valid for all of us. Even if you have underlying health issues and need to be under doctoral care, you would benefit significantly from walking for twenty minutes daily, eating one hundred grams of protein, and drinking 90 ounces of water daily. Yes, even fasting will help you, and most doctors are beginning to recommend it to more and more of their patients because of the health benefits.

When I followed up with Jen, she ate dinner and pushed her fast the following day. I was so proud of her. Can you guess why? Because treating herself compassionately and acknowledging her limitations was new territory for her. Before her first 30 days were over, Jen had already reached her 10-pound goal in 30 days and went on to lose 12 pounds. We never eliminated food groups, did no added time in the gym, longer fasts, or a supplement program. Jen has introduced herself to a system she can sustain for the rest of her life using basic scientific principles fueled with self-compassion and some awareness.

. . .

TAKING one bite-size piece at a time is counterintuitive for most.

"I have to be all in before I start" is a sentence I've heard repeatedly while helping women for the last five years. The Fasted Way Method proves that theory to be false, person by person.

EVERYBODY LOVES SOMETHING MINI

Do you remember when "mini" and "bite-size" started to grace the shelves in Target and Sephora and on menus in every restaurant? My favorite bite-size menu item has to be BJ's Brewhouse's "bazooka," a warm, freshly baked brownie cookie served in a pizza pan. No one ever wanted the Death By Chocolate, with a scoop of dark chocolate ice cream on top, and I would eat it all myself. When they introduced the mini trio, though, we could each pick a flavor, and I'm sure that saved me from a twenty-pound weight gain. What a fun phenomenon. If I can purchase something in a "mini size," it will always be an easy spend.

This societal trend could have influenced the "bite-size" approach woven into TFWM, but we'll leave Sephora and Pazookies behind this one. Will you take a moment to explore this core thought with me?

We are hard-wired to "go hard or go home." Most take it so far as to believe that if you don't take that approach23333, you won't get good results from your efforts. There are two problems with that theory. One, it is impractical. Your child is going to get a fever. You will attend a fun girl's weekend and drink bottomless mimosas. Emotional overwhelm will trigger hunger cues in your body, and you will binge eat the bag of potato chips. We've failed in the past because we try to pretend we are more robust than those inevitable circumstances. Just as dangerous, some of us have a moral belief that we are "stronger" and thus "better" if we can grit our teeth and rise above to "stay on track."

Good Lord. (Insert face palm emoji.)

Two, while you may see some results from your extreme approach, your body is a master adapter, and eventually, you will "plateau." In another section, we will talk about "plateauing," I will introduce an idea for you to chew on called "Set Point Theory." As a teaser, there is more to the story of the results you are or are not seeing than the food you eat and if you're exercising. Your emotions and nervous system play a huge part in your success.

To understand the "Bite-Size" approach used in The Fasted Way Method, you should know this part of Set Point Theory. Your nervous system, connected to your emotions, constantly searches for "safety." When we adopt extreme approaches to the felt mental and physical stress, it potentially hurts our feelings and, thus, hurts our nervous system. Your body will continue to hold onto fat because it is wired to make sure you don't starve and die. I'll explain it later, but "bite-size" is not extreme and doesn't signal those unsafe internal red flags to your emotions and nervous system. Then, the phenomenon happens where the scale goes down without learning to do one thousand burpees and only eat "a cube of cheese" to make an "Emily" throwback reference from The Devil Wear's Prada.

"When I feel like I'm going to faint, I just eat a cube of cheese," Emily Blunt's character says as Anne Hathaway's character "Andy" remarked how great she looked in her evening gown.

Does anyone remember the next scene with Emily's character? An injured Emily is binge eating jello and pudding cups from her hospital bed as the unfashionable "Andy" is taking Emily's spot in Paris Fashion Week, and Emily is in an emotional spiral downward.

Let's not be like Emily.

two

. . .

Why The Fasted Way Method Works

I remember when every menu, whether fast food or a sit-down dining restaurant, started including the calorie count of each item on their menu. It irritated me. 'I don't want to know how many calories I consume.' It felt intrusive. Underneath, I hadn't disconnected food choices from a moral attachment that if I ordered something with more calories, I was 'bad,' and if I ordered an item with two calories, I was 'good.' I had a drastic misunderstanding of calories and the role they play in our everyday lives.

Calories are essential for living, and your body needs calories to function. Your body takes the calories you give it through food and grows eyelashes. Feed your organs and aid your muscles in moving. More or less calories do not make you morally good or bad. In fact, as you read, I hope you begin to untangle yourself from the idea of 'good' and 'bad' around calories. To lose weight healthily and sustain your results over a long time, you will need to understand how calories work, what they are, and how to use them to your advantage.

food freedom

There she was, a very buff, blonde fitness influencer pouring a bowl of Reeses Puffs, shoveling spoonfuls into her mouth while milk flooded over the spoon back into the bowl. The caption talked about weight loss and food freedom. I'd never heard the term. I filed it away as one more marketing message that was intriguing and confusing, but the seed had been planted.

I can tell you now that food freedom does not happen without an understanding of calories and how they work. You can absolutely eat whatever you want, but most of us are ill-informed of the impending results of our food decisions. For this conversation about weight loss, let's look at calories from a deficit perspective while we lay out the entire method and how the pieces work together. Weight loss is nearly impossible without a deficit in your calorie intake.

CORE SCIENCE: Your body has to be in a calorie deficit to lose weight. Protein feeds your muscles and gives you a sense of fullness. Drinking enough water hydrates you and allows your body to flush out fat cells through urine and sweat. Moving your body is necessary for longevity and your overall health. Walking provides for the required calorie deficit without taking a hard toll on your body like other exercise approaches. Supplements can fill gaps and accelerate results.

Sounds easy. If you adopt this idea of asking good questions, you're already asking, how much protein, and how far do I walk? We'll get to that part. To adopt this approach into your life for the next 120 days and beyond, it's essential to understand why these scientific facts make the perfect scenario for you to get excellent results. Understanding how they all fit together will help you problem-solve if you feel stuck or stop seeing results.

bite size pieces

You start your Fasted Way journey with
1. One 8-hour fast per week.
2. Walking 1 mile per day.
3. Eating 100 grams of protein per day.
4. Drinking 90 ounces of water per day.
5. Optional supplements. I almost always supplement with a protein shake as my life is complete.

THAT WILL ENCOMPASS your first 30 days. You won't stay there, though. I hesitate to use the word "guarantee" because it's abused by sales reps who want you to feel safe to let go of your money. However, I don't know how you wouldn't see the scale decrease in your first 30 days if you consistently incorporate those five pillars into your daily life.

If you got the companion guide "Fast On Track Progress Tracker," you'll incrementally increase your fasting time frame, protein intake, and distance you walk. There are many reasons for this, but to keep it simple, this is why.

Core Science: Your body is a master adapter. (We will explain this more when we examine Set Point Theory.)

Because your body constantly tries to adjust to its desired comfort settings, we must take a bite-size, compassionate approach to weight loss methods. We also have to increase to get maximum results. Science doesn't change, but methods can and should be adaptable while keeping what we know is true.

method summary & a magic formula.

If you had a magic button to delete all of the great marketing, beautiful websites, and celebrity endorsements surrounding weight loss ideas, methods, and products - you would see a clear picture between aesthetics and hype versus science. What would be left for you to determine if something "works" would be results.

Results need no hype, and even if you had the ugliest website in the world, if the results were precise and defined, you would probably say, "Yes!"

Unfortunately, that button doesn't exist, and we are left with the ancient question, "Does that work?" And "Should I spend my money on that?"

Here are the scientific facts you can use as a compass for any product or program you're considering and why TFWM works.

scientific foundation & body of proof

1. Your body must be in a calorie deficit to burn fat and lose weight.
2. You have to move your body for overall health and weight loss.
3. Protein is king, and your body needs it to function.
4. Water is always the best drink, and it helps your body flush out fat through sweat and urine.
5. Supplements are great as " supplements" to your overall plan, but they will always fail if you cast them as the "star of the show" instead of a "supporting actor."

Mental and Emotional Approach:

1. A "Bite-size" incremental approach decreases mental and physical stress while getting results.

2. Any method has to be easily integrated into the rhythm of daily life. Most women have little room to learn something completely new.

3. The emotional boost of confidence fuels your desire to keep going.

4. Curiosity and asking good questions will always be your saving grace when encountering roadblocks, new ideas, or overwhelming circumstances.

The Fasted Way Method is built on the foundation of those five science-based facts while taking mental and emotional impact into account as well. It addresses putting our bodies into a calorie deficit. It factors in movement, focusing solely on walking for movement and exercise. Protein-powered weight loss works because we have to eat. Nutrition gets confusing because most don't know what to eat or how much to eat. This quickly leads to an overall feeling of defeat. When you connect once-per-week fasting fueled by protein, natural, long-lasting results show up quickly.

Yes, supplements are incredibly beneficial for filling our bodies with incredible nutrients we could be lacking from our food. Still, more than supplements alone will be needed to sustain results in the long term. This is the same for any of the other four categories.

Core Thought:

When we isolate a program or product as the sole proprietor for the weight of our health goals, we are destined to fail.

You have undoubtedly experienced this phenomenon. You are going back to the five pillars that make up the FWM: Calorie deficit, protein, water, movement, and supplements;

which one of the five have you addressed to help you get results? Have you ever addressed all five at the same time? Most people isolate one of those pillars and hope to see results in 4 weeks. There is no doubt putting a focus on any one of those key health components is a step in the right direction, but burnout, fatigue, and the demands of our daily lives have put the bar for results at what feels like unattainable heights.

BY REGULAR DIET and exercise standards, you'd have to be an Olympic pole vaulter to attain results with those methods.

When we solely focus on one health pillar to hold the entirety of our health goals, we set ourselves up to fail.

Welcome to your new normal. Your life is now fueled by science, self-compassionate goal setting with everything in bite-size pieces, and spreading the weight of your goals evenly over each necessary category. Now, you're set to run the marathon and are more likely to see long-term success.

i can't be the only one.

Have you ever signed up for an 8-week boot camp with a nutrition plan? You're excited and ready to go, but one of your kids throws up the night before it starts. The following day, your other kid throws up. By noon, your third kid has thrown up, and by 4:00 p.m., you think you're going to throw up.

The nausea, diarrhea, and vomiting continue for another 2-3 days, and then you catch it on the fifth day. By the time it's all said and done, 14 days have passed, and you've missed two weeks of boot camp. They've already progressed past the beginning to challenging workouts, and you don't even want to try to catch up.

This cycle is repeated many times, with a hundred different circumstances, and all of it adds up to you staying stuck and maybe even some weight gain because of stress eating.

What if you did something different that went along with the things you're already doing? If you could organize it just a smidge, and it didn't require you to do anything drastically different?

What you just read is not an ideal or a wish. It is the reality written in the pages you're about to read. Too often, women are derailed from their best-laid plans for growth or change because they don't account for the demands of their everyday lives.

LIBERTY LIBERATED GEN-Z

Liberty is a 22-year-old childcare professional who started The Fasted Way Method in August 2023. She lost seven pounds in her first week. Moving consistently through the method, she continued to see results. Then, as it does, life changed her daily rhythm. Someone very close to her passed away. Along with the influx of family togetherness that traditionally happens when a family experiences the loss of a loved one, there is also the emotional journey.

When she and I talked, I empathized with her loss and asked her how she was doing. Liberty wanted to talk about her Fasted Way journey. Amid life's tragedy, she felt frustrated that she wasn't staying "on track" with the new rhythm she'd been introduced to. She also feared losing the results she'd gotten.

I replied to her concerns, "Friend, this is why what we're

doing is different; life happens, and the method has to go along with it."

Then, I asked her which five pillars she felt comfortable focusing on. Walking, water, and protein were the three she mentioned. I cheered on her decision with encouragement.

"Thank you so much," she wrote back.

"That is what I love about you and your method. You don't push us to execute unrealistic perfection, and that is honestly the only reason I have been able to stay committed this long! Progress over perfection has become real in my life in the past few months, which is big."

That is the epitome of the Fasted Way Method, where compassion and science collaborate to support you.

definitions to know

The Fasted Way Method incorporates five pillars of biology with everyday living to help the Faster attain realistic results.

5 Pillars: Extended fasting, consuming water, movement, protein, and supplements.

DIY Weightloss: The idea that you should be able to implement and sustain anything you do for your health on your own. Phase 2 and Phase 3 of the 12-month method are in the online course "DIY Weight Loss."

Compassionate Goal Setting: Beyond typical goal setting, self-compassion asks, "What can I do in bite-size pieces that won't overwhelm me?"

Set Point Theory: Replacing "plateau" with this updated term, the Set Point Theory suggests your body has a set, internal "temperature" that works to keep your body regulated. Much like the thermostat in your house regulates the temperature in your home with pre-determined settings, your internal setting is connected to your *emotions and nervous system.*

CHECK *the back of the book for a code to access the on-demand video course that explains in depth what Set Point Theory is and how it is involved in your weight loss frustration.*

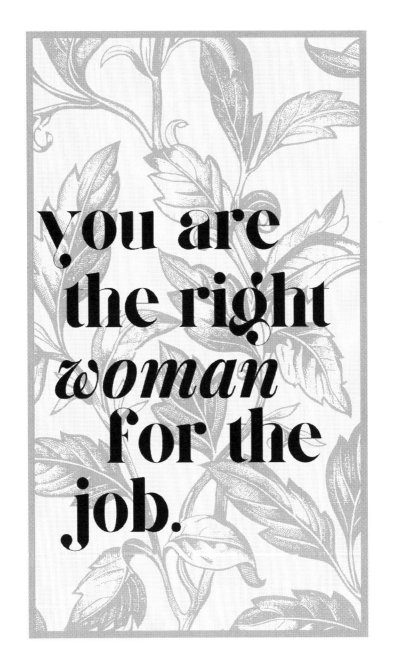

section
two

YOUR FIRST 8-HR FAST.

three

. . .

She Asked Me What? Most Asked Questions &
Please Keep Your Creamer.

T here is equal hesitation and amazement when I tell someone I didn't eat for a day and lost 40 pounds. I can see in their eyes the intrigue and horror. My weight loss results intrigue them, followed by shock. It started with something as simple as not eating for a day till dinner. The last two emotions are usually horror and doubt that they would be able to relinquish food for a day to jump-start weight loss. I can see the reflection of their favorite food in their pupils. I never put myself in the position of convincing.

I REMEMBER when my doctor suggested it to me the first time, I was horrified and wouldn't entertain the idea. It took two more unrelated exposures, talking about an 8-hour fast and autophagy fasting, for me to surrender to my doctor's recommendation. The same is true for you. It would be best if you saw this for yourself. This book won't convince you or employ hype to drive the point home. This method doesn't need hype. The Fasted Way Method stands on its merit, with results as proof. However, there is more to the story than simply abstaining from eating and seeing magical numbers pop up on the scale you haven't seen in a decade. A successful fast is just as much about how you prepare and end and your decisions the following day as it is about the actual time you're fasting.

the most asked questions

In August 2023, I posted on social media about my shock at the results I was seeing after listening to my doctor and incorporating an 8-hour fast. I didn't expect the flood of messages that followed. I asked a small group of women varying in age if they would be a part of a Beta Testing Group to see if I could teach them the method I'd created for myself to get them similar results. I am still shocked at how well it worked for many of them.

Their results fueled an accidental small business, and a complete career reroute for me, and their questions sent me deep into research to find answers. I'll address the most asked questions while we dive into what your 8-hour fast could look like.

THE MOST ASKED QUESTION IS, "Can I have _____." The words in the blank are usually "supplements/vitamins," "bone broth," "crystal light," or something to flavor your water. There is a straightforward way to answer all those inquiries, which isn't on a case-by-case basis. If "your blank" has any calories, the answer is "No!" The reason is that consuming that "thing" requires your digestive system to hit the "ON" switch going into digesting. The goal of your fast, regardless of length, is to put your digestive system in "Airplane Mode." The mechanics of fasting will be covered in a different chapter. Yes, it is essential, and you want to know the fireworks show is performing for you while you're fasting.

BLACK COFFEE & *A LOT OF WATER*

What I know is safe for keeping your digestive system auto-piloting smooth skies: black coffee and water when needed. You'll want to aim for 90 ounces daily, especially on the days you fast.

The type of coffee you choose is entirely up to you. One of the pillars of TFWM is that "all food" is morally neutral, meaning nothing is labeled as "good" or "bad." It will work if you prefer a cheap brand of coffee that you can get cheaply. If you grind the beans you picked in your backyard, that's great, too. This program works with all types of food choices.

One of the personal benefits for me has been overcoming an insane sugar habit triggered by a stress/trauma response. That leads me to a big question: "Can I have creamer?"

I'm a "little bit of coffee on the side to my creamer, whip, and chocolate syrup" gal. The thought of not having creamer in my coffee was not even an option I thought about or considered. I did get results from fasting while still putting creamer in my coffee. Until one day, I was out of creamer. Here's what happened.

One day, I may be able to fast without coffee. With two young kids at home and the demands of my everyday life, it is a compassionate choice to let myself have black coffee on fasting days. It gives me a boost of energy, suppresses my appetite, and doesn't break my fast. Giving up creamer was a complete accident. We get our groceries delivered (shout out to Instacart), and I'd just ordered groceries a few days before but didn't get creamer because I thought I had plenty. I didn't. I ran out.

I didn't "need" groceries except for creamer, and the order had a $35 minimum to get free delivery. Mentally, I couldn't justify spending $35 to get a $4.99 creamer. So, I drank my coffee black. It was disgusting, but it accomplished what I needed; I was less hungry. That was one year ago, and I haven't purchased creamer since then.

If you think I'm telling you to start drinking your black coffee, you may want to put this book in the trash now. I'm not. Creamer may be keeping you sane in your life, and you would've paid the $35 to get the creamer, and that's ok. This is a judgment-free process. I'm sharing because awareness is the first step to freedom. If you still drink creamer in your coffee, but you're not getting the results as fast as you think you should be, consider trying 8 hours without a creamer in your coffee.

Now, I drink my coffee cold. My Keurig makes my cheap cup of Community coffee. I promptly put ten ice cubes in it, and after it melts, I drink it in 2-5 minutes. As a mom, there isn't a lot of "sit" and "sip" time. Casually drinking a cup of coffee on a chilly fall morning will be a part of my life again one day. For now, I need to get it down. To the best of your ability, drink lots of water and drink black coffee when required.

DO I EXERCISE? *"Go hard or go home!"*

Regardless of what you have done in the past, whether you are a professional athlete or have never stepped foot in a gym, we need to ask this question based on who you are now, not who you used to be. The average human reading this book isn't asking that question. So, I will give this a big NO for needing to exercise on the days you're fasting.

If you are a former athlete or a "go hard or go home" kind of person, I'll tell you there are many opinions from experts about whether you should or shouldn't exercise while you fast and what types of exercise would be beneficial. If you are dead set on exercising while you fast, I'll encourage you to do your research.

I would ask you, "How often do you rest?" By rest, I mean mentally and physically. How often do you laugh without being prompted by something you saw on your phone or TV? As I've coached and listened to many different types of men and women through their health goals, I can tell you that your desire to "go hard" and avoid resting has much more to do with your emotional capacity and your ability to sit with yourself; the parts of you that you can suppress with "going," and a "good sweat sesh." Even good things done with the wrong motives can quickly become the "wrong thing."

Something I was genuinely worried about was being "hangry." I didn't realize that my lifestyle of high sugar consumption left me with a lot of nausea and headaches when I didn't eat. I thought it was because I had a high metabolism. It is higher than the average, but glucose spikes were the cause of my insane appetite, and I didn't know until one day when I was fasting... (cue the going back in time harp sounds.)

I have a son with special needs, and he can move and run very fast. On a day I was fasting, he jumped on his bike, didn't want to stay on our street, and went to the park while ignoring my yells to "Stop!" As I ran in full sprint after him, I thought: "Am I going to vomit from hunger after this?" It was a valid question because throwing up and exercising were equally a part of my experience whenever I went to the gym in my 20s. It was something I was afraid of. It is incredible what our bodies can do when given the right tools.

I didn't vomit, and I did catch my runaway son. I had no adverse reactions other than a lot of sweat. I was fine. "You're ok!" I was shockingly saying to myself. There are no guarantees of what your fasting journey will reveal about YOU. Coming to the "fasting" table for weight loss is where many are starting this conversation, but beyond that initial desire is an incredible journey of discovery introducing your-self to you. That is the real reward.

MY OPINION: **Do not exercise on your fasting days. Prioritize rest. But if you have to chase your speedy kid, you'll be just fine.**

four

. . .

Can You Make It Till Dinner?

The first four hours of your fast will be spent digesting what's already in your system. Your body will burn what it already has for fuel and energy, and the types of foods you've been eating leading up to that fast will be very apparent. When I started to get nauseous, I realized I'd been overconsuming carbs and "celebration food." To help. Yourself feel good, do these three things 48 hours before your fast:

1. Eat 100 grams of protein each two days leading up to your first 8-hour fast. No matter what you've been eating before this moment, consuming more protein will answer MANY questions your body has about weight loss.
2. Eat good fats. Our bodies and brains need fat, and it is easier to get in with paying attention. Ensure you get the "The Good Fat Life with A Side Of Protein" for a list of fats you probably already have in your house. A QR code at the back of this

book will take you to a website to download a PDF with a suggested meal plan.

3. Last, have your "dinner" prepped the day before your fast. You'll also want to go to the grocery store before the day of your fast.

4. Be aware of how often you reach for food that isn't a protein, a vegetable, a fruit, or beverages you gravitate to other than water or coffee. We aren't an elimination program, and you will not get a list of foods you need to get rid of to be successful. Awareness, though, is your best friend. Eating more protein and food higher in fat will help you feel full. So, potentially, you won't reach for the other stuff as much as you usually would. Even if you do and decide to eat your favorite thing - IT'S OK! Being aware, taking good mental notes, or writing it down in the back of your "Fast On Track" tracker is a great idea.

day of fast

- *Wake up in the morning and consume water.*
- *After a few hours, have a cup of black coffee or green*
- *tea. Do not consume coffee or green tea right in the*
- *mornlng. Utilize thcsc only when you start feeling*
- *hungry. When you're ready to break your fast like steak or salmon.*
- *Include a non-starchy vegetable and a starchy vegetable for your carbs. Drizzle it with a good-*

sized tablespoon of olive or avocado oil for bonus fats. After
- *Eight 8 hours of fasting, you will notice that even a small*
- *meal is enough to fill your stomach.*
- *Make sure that the meal is very high in fatty protein;*
- *Otherwise, you will defeat the purpose of fasting all day.*

day after fast

1. *Weigh right when you wake up.*
2. *Have your 100 grams of protein pre-planned. A lot of hard work on your fasting day can be undone simply because you didn't plan. Don't worry about any other food groups. We'll cover fats and carbohydrates. For now, focusing on prioritizing protein will be enough of an adjustment and will keep your progress moving forward.*
3. *Walk 1-3 miles. You can walk 1 or 3 miles daily, depending on your current mobility. We'll discuss this more when we discuss movement.*
4. *Water, water, water! If it helps, get a designated drinking cup that visually reminds you to drink from it.*
5. *If you're taking supplements or using a program, you can resume taking whatever supplements you're used to. Protein powder or pre-made protein drinks are excellent supplements for your day.*

6. *Plan three more 8-hour fasts for the next three weeks, exactly like you did. Try to stick to the same day each week, but if it ends up being a different day, that's okay.*

sample of 8-hr fast schedule

- SUNDAY Last meal - 8 pm
- Sleep - 11 pm
- MONDAY
- Wake up - 7 am
- Drink water - 7 am
- Drink water - 9 am
- Drink green tea - 11 am
- Drink water - 1 pm
- Drink water - 3 pm
- Drink coffee - 5 pm
- Eat Dinner - 6 pm
- Sleep - 11 pm

Drink water to stay hydrated as and when required. Shown above is just an example.

the scale & true chat calories

(We won't count them, but we must discuss them.)

———

IF YOU DON'T OWN a scale, or the one you have needs new batteries, you will want to have that ready. In my 20s, I sold vitamins and weight loss programs through Advocare.

Over and over, I told women to "put their scale in the driveway and back over it with their car." It was the worst advice I could have given. In 2021, I was training to run a half-marathon with a fantastic coach. Once a week, she would bring a scale so we could track my weight loss progress. I learned so much about myself.

For some women, the scale has been used as a weapon against their bodies. A few women I've coached couldn't bring themselves to step on the scale because of the emotional flood of guilt and shame when the digital numbers would pop up in flashing digital horror. If that is how you feel, don't step on the scale. You'll be able to feel the bloating dissipate, your clothes will start to feel different, and your energy should increase. If you still can't bring yourself to step on the scale, please seek help and allow a professional thera-pist to walk you through the emotions that come up for you.

The scale is one of many tools your body can use to give you feedback. I had a meltdown in December of 2021 when I saw the scale increase by three pounds. I was aware I wasn't having a normal response, but I also didn't try to tell myself I shouldn't be having that response or my feelings were wrong or bad. There is always a reason we react the way we do. I have been equally excited and frustrated as I've stepped on the scale. Sometimes, I "feel" fat to then step on the scale and see a small number to realize that my "feeling" was not reality in a positive way. Other times, the number flashing back at me has sparked curiosity.

I start to go back and analyze my activity over the past week. Your "Fast On Track Progress Tracker" is a fantastic companion for this very example. We cannot know every-thing, but we can eliminate so much guesswork with aware-ness and educating ourselves on what to do.

The scale is feedback. Without feedback, you can't problem-solve. It is not reflective of your value as a person. The number on the scale does not make you "bad" or "good." You are important because you are a living, breathing human deserving of dignity regardless of physical appearance.

Before your 8-hour fast, weigh yourself and write that number in your tracker. The morning after your fast, weigh again, write down that number, and note your loss.

more or less

When you weigh yourself, remember that number reflects your whole person, even the weight of your hair. "Losing weight" is not just losing fat; you'll see that reflected on the scale. Losing water weight is not just "water." Sodium and carbohydrates hold water and are stored in the body as glycogen. Glycogen is your body's go-to fuel source. When you start a fast or even in the first 30 minutes of exercise, your body burns glycogen for fuel.

Digestive bloat and backed-up waste in your system, otherwise known as "bloat," is one of the first benefits you'll see from your first few fasts. Often, people will see a 2-5 pound loss from their first 8-hour fast. Some of that could be fat loss. More than likely, it's your body burning the fuel you've been giving it. Gut health is a primary focus in fasting, and we aren't adding anything to your daily intake to help your gut. Most people have enough tacos and wedding cake stored In their gut to last through 12 months of fasting without needing to add anything extra for gut health. Your body knows what to do.

Fat loss is the long-term goal, and depending on how much weight you have to lose will determine the numbers you see reflected on the scale after a fast. If you have over one hundred pounds to lose, you will probably see a five or more pounds loss from your first fast. As you follow the 120-Day Fasting Schedule in this book and the downloadable PDF, it is reasonable to say you could lose over fifteen pounds in your first 30 days of following this method. That is how ready your body is to release the excess weight it carries. Your body is not meant to have excess. The excess looks different for everyone, but your body will respond significantly as you use the right tools.

If you are within twenty pounds of your body's ideal weight, it will probably take ten to fifteen weeks to see the overall results you're looking for. There are a few reasons, but the biggest is Set Point Theory. Your body wants to keep you safe. You are training your body to live and adapt to the world you've created through your emotional responses, eating habits, sleep routine, and relationships. While this method is beyond incredible, no matter how much weight you have to lose, the last ten pounds will require focus, determination, and discipline. As you adjust to a new routine, incorporate new supports for your nervous system, and eat fewer Oreos and a little more salmon, your body will find rest and respond how you want it to.

I've heard, and you've probably heard, that safe weight loss is 1-2 pounds per week. As you follow The Fasted Way Method, you'll see that reflected in the results you get. A condensed calorie deficit is the main component allowing this system to work well. When talking about "calories," there are three choices: you can be in a deficit, you can be in maintenance, or you can be in surplus. You've been bouncing between those three categories and unaware of what's happening.

Every person has a certain amount of calories to eat daily to live. Your organs need to function, your hair needs to grow, your brain needs to function, and your heart needs to beat.

Food is the primary way our bodies accomplish LIVING. Do you know what your maintenance calories are? It's based on your height and your weight. You also factor in your activity level and workouts into those numbers. If you have a low exercise (this doesn't include NEAT: Non-exercise Activity Thermogenesis, which refers to calories burned doing everyday regular movement that isn't exercise.)

For most of us, the only time we talk about calories is when we want to lose weight. For years, I wanted to gag when someone would mention "counting calories" because it felt like deprivation, and I never saw anyone maintain their results by simply cutting calories. What are your thoughts about calories? Do you immediately picture all the food you're not allowed to have or a menu with the amount of calories next to each item?

When you go into a calorie deficit, you eat less than your body needs, hoping it will burn fat for fuel to replace the calories you are not eating. It doesn't mean your body needs less to operate, but stored body fat will bridge the gap. This is a scientific fact that being in a calorie deficit is one of the only ways to see the scale number decrease.

The problem, however, is that most women already have a calorie deficit but don't realize it. Some women have been underrating for decades and don't know. This is horrendous for our hormones, our sleep, our moods, and our overall health. So, when you go to "lose weight" and someone tells you to be in a "calorie deficit," how can you eat less than what you're already eating when you're barely eating as it is? Suppose you regularly skip significant meals and can't immediately tell me how much protein you eat daily. In that case, I can almost guarantee you are underrating and eating less than fifty grams of protein. Ask me how I know... Because I've yet to have a conversation with a woman I'm coaching who wants to lose weight and is eating enough protein, and her eating is regulated and on a routine.

Eating in "surplus" calories is more than your body needs. Often, this is our weekend fun or holiday eating. While many condemn that type of behavior, saying, "I've fallen off the wagon" or adopting "cheat meals" or "cheat days," I think that is a horrible mentality to adopt. I'm not a dog and don't reward myself for "good eating" with "treats." Life is meant to be enjoyed, and food is one of the ways we partake in this globally accepted ritual. In every country on our planet, each culture has a practice of gathering around the table. The table is where laughter, connection, and community happen. We are hard-wired to need those social connections with our families and friends, and it revolves around food on the table.

Can you imagine gathering without food? Have you ever been to a Thanksgiving where the turkey was replaced with tofu or fish in an attempt to be more "healthy?" It is disheartening. If you are someone who is regularly depriving yourself of food, then binging all the "good food," slow down, and pay attention to the emotions connected to this eating cycle. How do you feel emotionally and physically when you decide to restrict? How do you feel emotionally and physically when you choose to eat in surplus?

Don't ask those questions in the place of "I'm doing something wrong" or assessing because you're going to change all the "bad behaviors." No, this is something of much higher importance. Observe yourself objectively without judgment. Eating in surplus often brings emotions of fulfillment, satisfaction, and contentment. Yes, when we overdo it, there can also be misery, indigestion, and diarrhea for my ice cream indulgent lactose intolerant friends. But for a moment, let's pretend you enjoy surplus eating at your favorite restaurant with a burger, fries, and a milkshake. How do you feel after? Happy?

Those emotions are directly connected to your nervous system. Our nervous systems have many functions, but one of the higher functions is controlling memory, thinking, reasoning, learning, and regulating emotions. The brain partners with the signals from the nervous system, allowing creativity, decision-making, and problem-solving.

I'm not a scientist or nutritionist and do not give medical or therapeutic advice. I am a researcher solving my problems, and what I've discovered about the nervous system and its connections to our emotions through the brain has left me excited and shaken. Your nervous system and brain control autonomic functions like heart rate, blood pressure, and hormone release. So, what does this have to do with your burger, fries, and milkshake?

Would you agree that eating your favorite foods makes you feel emotionally satisfied as your body feels full and satisfied? A sense of contentment after a favorite meal is intrinsic to human nature. Simultaneously, picture Monday morning after a "binge weekend"? Imagine the foods you're going to force yourself to eat. What are they?

Imagine the food you're going to miss. What are they? I bet you spend most of the week looking forward to the weekend again. Why? Because that burger is calling your name, but deeper, it's the sense of fullness and contentment, both emotionally and physically, that we are hard-wired to have that you are missing in your every day. Calculating calories will not be a part of the 120-day fasting timeline. You will focus on eating 100 grams of protein daily, an 8-hour fast once a week that builds to longer fasts, and walking 1 mile daily.

However, for your sanity and calorie awareness, we will "indulge" the conversation of calories a little further.

"have you met templeton, the rat?"

You have more than likely read the famous book "Charlotte's Web" by famed author E.B. White or seen the original cartoon. Templeton the Rat is the character you love to hate in the story. Templeton is a rat doing ratty things who continues to get roped into aiding Charlotte the Spider to save Wilbur the Pig from being Christmas dinner. Templeton is coaxed into helping as Charlotte strategically aligns Wilbur's well-being with Templeton's survival.

In one of the conversations, Charlotte asks for Templeton's help as he can venture in and out of places where none of the other animals can. In need of words to weave into her web, Charlotte sends a complaining Templeton off to find a word, and he begrudgingly complies. The strip of paper he comes back with says, "CRUNCHY." Well, even if you haven't read the story, you would probably agree that using the word "crunchy" in conjunction with a pig only brings up memories of perfectly cooked bacon and is not reasonable grounds for making a plea to spare the little pig's life letting him keep his bacon.

Charlotte asks him to go out again, and you can imagine the rat's disgusted refusal even though the overflow of Wilbur's feed trough is the rat's primary food source. In the 1973 adaption of the book, the Goose speaks up and puts starvation squarely into Templeton's view.

"Why should I worry about Wilbur?" Templeton asks.

"You'll worry alright when winter comes," the Goose responds. "If Wilbur is killed and his trough stands empty, you'll grow so thin we'll be able to look right through your stomach and see objects on the other side."

Terrified, Templeton looks back at Charlotte and says, "Ok, Charlotte, what did you have in mind?"

Later in the book, Wilbur is headed to the fair, and Templeton's help is needed again, but he doesn't want to oblige. Charlotte the Spider appeals to his indulgent nature as we respond to that weekend cheat meal. She reminds him of all the food he'll be able to gorge himself on. Templeton gets the message and fulfills his obligation, and when the lights go out at the fair, he heads out for a rat's smorgasbord feast of leftover popcorn, half-eaten hot dogs, and cotton candy. If you've never seen it, you should watch the clip on YouTube.

So many of us live the same way: somewhere between starvation, looking forward to being able to eat the food we love and overindulging to the point of misery. What makes the guilt of Monday morning worth it? The momentary feeling of contentment and happiness when your mouth is full of your favorite tastes and flavors (that's your nervous system).

We shouldn't want to take out all joy from food. Food is good, and we should enjoy it. Emotions of delight will always come up when you eat something you love, and the feeling of disgust will undoubtedly arise when you eat something you loathe. You will never be able to separate those inner wirings. It is a part of your human fabric. What we can work through is eating in excess to our detriment. While we won't ever separate food and emotions, we won't be able to delete the scientific and nutritional facts of overindulgence. What that looks like, though, is different for each person. Start by discovering the maintenance calories needed for your activity level, height, and weight. Experience what life is like when you know about eating in those calories. Because your nervous system, emotions, hormones, and brain are connected, your brain starts associating certain foods with negative emotions.

You can begin to re-write your food story without eliminating what you love, and The Fasted Way Method is the path to weight loss while enjoying food. Are you ready for the secret?

fasted calories & protein dreams

Hopefully, you've accepted the "calorie deficit" truth and checked that box in the mental checklist and toolbox of info we're building. The fact of calorie deficit is unchanging, but the method by which you get into a calorie deficit can change and should adapt as we discover more about the body through scientific discovery.

Fasting is the method that allows you to be in a calorie deficit in a condensed period versus the traditional method. Traditional weight loss wants you to be in a calorie deficit every day. Few programs tell you how long that should last, though, and years of living in an unknown daily calorie deficit is part of why many of us are in the weight loss boat. That isn't even mentioning the havoc underrating nutrients like fat is having on our hormones, leading to all sorts of crazy issues.

In the first 30 days of your fasting timeline, you will complete four 8-hour fasts, focusing one day per week on the schedule we covered. When you fast in this way, you accomplish your body's need for a calorie deficit to jump-start weight loss. The best part, however, is that we don't stay there, and food is not the only way you're going to burn calories. You can accomplish more in one 8-hour fast per week than all the years you've lived in an unknown calorie deficit.

Even better, you aren't eliminating anything. Instead, we focus on what we ARE going to eat, leaving room for what we want. This will be covered more deeply when we talk about protein, but the power of focusing on protein as prioritizing it FIRST in your daily food intake is where your body will show off what it's capable of.

Circling back to the core idea that fuels The Fasted Way Method - is it the fasting that is the star? Or is it the protein? Or maybe it's walking, which we'll talk about for movement. Or perhaps all these pieces work simultaneously in harmony, giving your body what it needs, that is, the show's star.

LET'S PUT IT IN A TORTILLA, which is a fun way of saying 'Here's your conclusion':

Nervous system regulation is imperative for overall health and is closely connected to our body's ability to lose weight. For more research, look up Dr. Nicole LePera's 'The Holistic Therapist' and 'The Garden Within' by Dr. Anita Phillips on Audible.

Calories have three categories: maintenance, deficit, and surplus, and we are actively working through those three areas knowingly or unknowingly. None of them are wrong. Not knowing these categories exist, though, can be detrimental. Look up calorie intake according to your height and weight for further research.

The Fasted Way Method allows you to work within a condensed timeframe to accomplish your body's calorie deficit needs. It also demonstrates the power of prioritizing protein and does not teach eliminating or removing food you enjoy. Scan the QR codes in the back to get this book's companion tracker and goal-setting journal.

"We *have demonized* carbs, down played the power of protein. and left women with nothing but a plate of *starvation and guilt.*"

section
three

THE INTERNAL LENS
& SCIENCE OF COMPASSION

five

. . .

The Science Of Compassion

Are you familiar with this quote: *"Great things never came from comfort zones?"—Anonymous*.

I imagine the same person who wrote this post didn't sign their name for fear of getting their house toilet papered by a group of women who'd been awake, breast-feeding all night. I would bet they never wore pantyhose and had a tampon dry up without a replacement at your kid's soccer game with no bathroom in sight. If you are a female, you could write a list of uncomfortable areas in your life that are non-negotiable parts of your everyday life.

Life is full of discomfort. Your plan to lose weight shouldn't be one of those places. Would it be safe to assume your life isn't going to stop so you can solely focus on your health? Most days, you probably have time to feed your tiny humans, much less a meal plan for yourself. Am I right? We are navigating schedules and laundry; some take care of aging family members while juggling full-time jobs. Then, we scroll social media and see the garage of messages coming at us in machine gun style about everything you should be doing to lose weight.

. . .

IT IS OVERWHELMING.

COMPASSION for yourself is the heart behind addressing the problem you just read above. It is unrealistic from a logistical view, cruel from an emotional view, and detrimental from a scientific biological view. Compassionate goal-setting has to become your new compass for determining your weight loss goals. Before deciding on any approach, you should slow down and take inventory of yourself.

BEFORE WE HIT GO

There are two resources already created that I want to reference and that are available as companions to this book. "Just Don't" is an interactive goal-setting journal for your weight loss journey. You'll love it because it will guide you through the process of compassionate goal setting with questions and fill in the blanks so you can know yourself better. It's the process I developed for myself that helped me lose the forty pounds I gained through binge eating sugar. Scan the QR code at the back of this book to get yours as a companion to this section.

Second is a free mini course called "Ain't Your Mama's Fast." You'll learn about 'Set Point Theory' and why the "Go Hard Or Go Home" you've taken in the past has led you straight down the path to weight loss burnout. It will also show you an alternative route and go back to compassionate goal setting for your weight loss journey. Scan the QR code on the back of this book, and you can watch it immediately.

half-marathon hopes & costco size nutella

Desperation can create a hunger for change. However, if desperation is also attached to the worth you see in yourself, you will miss the bigger picture and fail. Let me paint it for you.

When I say I had a "sugar addiction," I need to paint a clear picture of what that looked like. A perfect example was the February I was hiding in my pantry eating spoonfuls of Nutella. It was Valentine's Day weekend, and I'd ordered Nutella from Costco to make Nutella heart-shaped pancakes. Well, you and I know Costco only sells everything in double canisters in more ounces than anyone needs. I made the pancakes, but after 24 hours, one-and-a-half of the containers I'd consumed with a spoon while hiding in my pantry. That, my friends, is not just a lack of self-control. I'd been facing debilitating depression that fall, with many days spent sleeping because I didn't know what else to do. I'd considered medication because I was struggling to function and complete basic tasks.

What I would later learn, thanks to educators who see the value of creating content through social media, was that binge eating was a trauma response. It was how I coped with stress and lived through domestic abuse during most of my childhood. It wasn't as simple as "lacking discipline and self-control." If you are someone who has faced any abuse in a single event or extended event, you cannot classify your body and your emotions. They are linked, and that will never change. We can continue forcing ourselves into a "Boot Camp" style weight loss or exercise program to move our bodies to do what we're demanding, or we can choose something different. We can choose *compassion*.

With the Nutella canister in one hand and the spoon in my mouth, I looked down at the half-gone contents and immediately realized what I was doing. I threw the second canister away and made a mental note: "That wasn't normal."

I didn't know then that I would accumulate all the necessary tools over the next three years to find "normal." Here are just a few I saw as I am now actively looking for a trauma therapist as well:

- I am learning how to regulate my nervous system with non-food and non-spend stimulants. You can follow Dr. Nicole LePera, "The Holistic Psychologist," on social media.
- Any books by Suzanne Stabile explaining the interworkings of the enneagram.
- Working with macro coaches as I learned about Reverse Dieting.
- I was a great running and lifting coach who taught me proper form.
- The EvolveYou app for lifting programs, and following the creator Krissy Cela for continuing education about lifting.
- "Resilient" by John Eldridge.
- My doctor: I saw him monthly for a weight management program and accountability.
- "How To Keep House When You're Drowning" by KC Davis.

AS I'VE ADDRESSED my whole person and the needs of each part of me, success in weight loss has quickly become a side dish. It was the key, opening the door to a more extensive conversation. Weight loss is not one-size-fits-all. I'm glad you are reading this book if you've struggled to know where to start. As you continue your journey, return to the list above if you are trying to find your next steps.

HALF-RUNNING

My answer to binging Nutella was not to slow down and examine compulsive habits linked to deeper emotional issues. No, I decided to run a half-marathon. I'd lost ten pounds a few years before by running my first 5k. I thought, "If I run longer, I'll lose more weight." I was so wrong.

Have you ever watched someone train for a 5k or half-marathon, see their weight loss results, and think, "I'll try that." That was my thought, too. I found an incredible coach to help me strength train and run my first half-marathon, and what I learned from her was invaluable. But four months after running 13.1 miles for the first time, I hit exercise burnout. After nine months of training, I had not seen the results I thought I was going to. Instead of a daily walk or run to help with stress, I returned to my default settings: impulsive spending and eating vast amounts of sugar until the entire party-size bag of mini York Peppermint Patties was gone. I wanted to numb my life and everything I couldn't control. I saw the problems and issues sucking the oxygen out of my life but felt powerless to create positive change.

"Netflix and chill" with a party size of whatever I could get delivered the fastest became my everyday routine. After fighting through depression, binge eating sugar, and trying to compensate with exercise to force my body to lose weight; it was time to address the "why" behind the habits that were sabotaging my weight loss plans. I relied on exercise and supplements to do all the "heavy lifting," hoping that these two tools that had worked in my 20s and early 30s would work in my late 30s, but my body said, "No!"

YOUR NUTELLA MOMENT

What you just read was a nonjudgmental, curious approach to the entire answer to my weight loss gain. You can do that for yourself, too. Instead of segmenting your life and denying emotional impact, look at the whole picture. Here's a way you can do that.

Close your eyes and go to the moment you thought, "I have to do something about this." Was it wearing everyday clothes, realizing your "big clothes" were feeling small? Maybe seeing your reflection in the mirror before you got in the shower? Do you have that moment in your mind? Can you see it?

Now, go back four months. What did the whole picture of your life look like? You should grab a piece of paper and pen and write it down chronologically if the image in your mind is fuzzy. You may need to go back six months, a year, or five years. I don't want to make excuses for habits that lead to unhealthiness in our bodies (not just the number on the scale - unhealthy in every area of our lives.) I do want to help you create compassion for yourself. Recognizing trigger responses that lead to decisions not aligned with our long-term goals and putting support in place when those inevitable moments surface has to become part of your weight loss plan.

If not, you plan to fail.

What I want you to see are patterns. Instead of looking at those patterns through emotions like shame or guilt, look at them objectively. Be curious about you. Allow yourself to be human. Being "human" acknowledges that we are mind, body, soul, and spirit. Disconnecting where we are in our physical bodies from our minds, will, and emotions means no matter what we do to attain health, we will ultimately fail. The trees are linked, and you cannot unlink them.

You can ignore the connection, but you cannot delete the fact. We demand perfection from our bodies without considering the state of our mind and soul and its direct effect on our physical bodies.

If we fail to slow down and consider the connection, we will always find ourselves in the same place.

the mind-body connection: muscle, fat, & your bmi

It's important to note a few things about fat, muscle, and overall weight loss. You've already seen a breakdown of what happens internally when you fast, but you need to know that you are losing total overall body mass, not just fat. Starting a weight loss journey doesn't allow you to choose where the weight will come from. As we've already covered, "losing weight" encompasses your entire person: fat, muscle, intestinal waste, water weight retention from overconsuming carbs, and yes, even your hair. When you step on the scale, the number reflects everything in your body, not just how much fat your body holds.

What I've learned that I wish I had known years ago is to measure your overall BMI, but more importantly, your muscle mass. What I couldn't track as I was strength training and running long distances was the transition of fat to muscle. It's called Body Composition.

Body composition is an essential measure of overall health, reflecting the balance between fat and lean muscle mass. When we talk about muscle "replacing" fat, we describe a process where, through intentional movement and strength training, your body gradually builds muscle while reducing fat stores. It's essential to recognize that this doesn't always lead to a significant drop in weight but rather a shift in how your body looks and feels. Muscles are denser than fat, so even if the number on the scale stays the same, your body may appear leaner and more toned.

This transformation is a positive sign that you're becoming more robust and healthier from the inside out. With more muscle, your body burns more calories, even at rest, boosting your metabolism and helping sustain long-term health. It's not just about numbers or appearances— improving your body composition enhances how you move, feel, and live, giving you more incredible energy and confidence in your daily life.

It is vital to approach this process with patience and compassion for your body, as these changes take time and care. Each step forward reflects your progress toward a healthier, more resilient version of yourself.

Because the general population of women trying to "be smaller" is confused about many fundamentals, you have no context to compare that number to when you look at the scale.

Also, long-distance cardio breaks down muscle; it doesn't feed muscle or allow you to look "lean." I wanted my legs to have shape, and after nine months of training and running further than ever, I wasn't seeing any muscular definition. I also wasn't seeing my legs decrease in size. Part of the problem was that I didn't have all the into, so I saw the scale increase and quit altogether. I was so defeated.

We'll cover this more when we discuss protein and walking, but getting an idea of your muscle mass is more important than your overall Body Mass Index. Some gyms have the technology to measure muscle mass. Also, it is essential to note that if you work out and do not eat the correct calories to compensate for the exercise, you will not see the results you are looking for.

The macro coaches I worked with were worth every penny I paid. However, the average American woman doesn't have $300-$500 monthly to get your macros customized weekly. Simultaneously, when I tried to figure out how the coaches calculated my macros, they were hesitant to share or wouldn't answer my direct questions.

When I went to the internet to try and figure out what my calories should be, it was like Alice chasing the White Rabbit down a never-ending hole. I kept saying, "Weight loss shouldn't be this hard." Forty pounds have been lost using this method I created for myself. I can tell you it isn't as hard as we've made it.

For now, I want to help you jump-start weight loss by employing a calorie deficit through fasting and protecting and feeding your muscles by increasing your protein. That sounds pretty simple. Simple and easy mean different things. I aim to simplify this simple system with the right tools and under-standing the whole process.

THERE'S MORE TO THE STORY

Excess fat in the body is a widely known danger to our health. However, the risks of females losing muscle mass and the preventable diseases connected to increasing muscle are not equally amplified as an alternative to obsessing over how lousy obesity is.

Please remember from the section: Science is a living, breathing thing, and humans constantly discover it.

In 2013, a research paper was produced detailing a new metric called the "BRI" Body Roundness Index. Lead researcher Dr. Jose M. Guedes partnered with a team of scientists to find a better metric than BMI for measuring total body fat. Their goal was to highlight prevention methods for diseases connected to obesity.

Three years later, in 2016, Japanese professor and researcher Yoshinori Ohsumi was recognized for discovering how genes and the body's molecular structure benefitted from"Autophagy." Ohsumi won the Nobel Peace Prize in Physiology and Medicine that year.

However, his work was likely influenced by a Belgian biochemist, Christian de Duve, who discovered autophagy in the 1960's. As we already covered ['ol/k,πæ]\k, "Autophagy" is an internal mechanism each of our bodies possesses for our cells to degrade and recycle damaged parts of the cell itself.

Science is catching up to the rest of us in 2024, with voices like Dr. Mindy Pelz and famed actor Chris Hemsworth championing "autophagy" for all the benefits you've been reading about here.

You are likely reading this book because you want to lose weight. That is important. We want to live longer and have a better quality of life. Carrying more weight than your body is designed to can impede those long-term goals, while the correct fat and muscle ratio can enhance it. The story doesn't stop there, though. Your body is capable. Knowing that brilliant scientists are working on research to help us achieve our full potential is encouraging. We may not learn about it for ten years, but applying this method is a fantastic place to

six

. . .

The Most Unboring Science You'll Ever Read.

W hile frolicking down the TikTok rabbit hole, searching for that elusive "decompress mom-brain time," I was jolted out of my scroll trance. There he was—Thor, the mighty god of thunder, not wielding Mjölnir (his mighty hammer for those that haven't seen any of the movies) but instead chatting casually about the health merits of fasting. Can you imagine? The juxtaposition was so surreal I was utterly hooked! After reading through this science, you will be too.

I am an avoider of pain, all pain: physical, emotional, relational...Burpees and Broad Jumps fall in this category; I won't do them!! If it involves pain, I am probably going to stay far away. I have to be very intentional when facing pain and discomfort. I draw courage from focusing on the promised benefit of the painful process. The payoff has to be worth it. The second place I draw courage from is understanding why I'm doing what I'm doing and researching the process. Knowledge fuels belief. Belief fuels faith. Faith drives action. So, all I have to say to you is 'Welcome back to Biology 101."

The best place to start is understanding the physical benefit of extending fasting; there is a lot more happening than just 'losing weight."

When I started extended fasting in 2023, I didn't have the list you were about to read. As I began researching to help the August Beta group understand, I discovered science that brought language to what I was experiencing. I experienced the benefit first and then found the list later. You're getting a tricky start, so there is no question you will be successful. This list helped me finally accomplish my first 24-hour fast and pushed me to longer fasts. Get ready because we'll use some scientific terms but make it as painless as possible.

"FIVE SECRET BENEFITS *to Fasting from Food You Had No Idea Existed."*

It will put your body into a **Caloric Deficit***:* Fasting for a day significantly reduces your overall calorie intake for that week. This caloric deficit can help restart weight loss by forcing your body to tap into stored fat for energy. We will talk about this more, but when you take less, your body is forced to use what it already has (stored body fat) for energy.

Metabolic Flexibility: I know, I know, the last time you were able to use the word "flexible" when applied to your body was in high school. But, girl, you've got a flex you didn't know about. Regular fasting can improve your body's metabolic flexibility, so it becomes better at switching between burning glucose (sugar) and burning fat for energy. This can help prevent your metabolism from slowing down during prolonged periods of calorie restriction and, again, tells your body to use stored body fat for energy.

Insulin Sensitivity: Fasting can improve insulin sensitivity, making it easier for your body to regulate blood sugar levels.

When your insulin sensitivity increases, your body is less likely to store excess calories as fat.

Hormone Regulation: Fasting can impact hormones like ghrelin (the hunger hormone) and leptin (the hormone that signals fullness), potentially reducing appetite and helping you control your calorie intake.

Psychological Reset: Breaking through a weight loss plateau can also be a mental challenge. A day of fasting can serve as a mental reset, helping you regain focus and motivation for your weight loss journey.

It's important to note that fasting may not be suitable for everyone, and it's essential to consult with a healthcare professional or registered dietitian before starting any fasting regimen.

FOR A MOMENT, I want to come back and highlight "Insulin Sensitivity.' I didn't know when I was fasting that I was giving my body the tool it finally needed to kill and bury a life-long sugar addiction. From time to time, it tries to 'come back from the dead,' but I've been able to recognize the response in my body when I have the compulsion to devour the whole bag of York Peppermint Patties - party-size - not kidding! I know now the physical response my body is having is from trauma and is a learned behavior. If it had not been for fasting, I wouldn't have been able to recognize the feeling and put non-food supports in place to continue giving my body the right tools that don't derail my progress. It all came back to insulin sensitivity.

Fasting doesn't mean deprivation – it's an intentional choice to give your body a break from digestion and to tap into your body's natural healing abilities. I asked, "Why does my body need a break from digestion?"

NOTE: Different people have contacted me asking about specific medical issues and if my actions would be safe for them. A big one has been if it's secure while breast-feeding. Checking with your doctor is always the place to start. More health practitioners are recommending extended fasting to their clients. Also, do your research. Find others facing your specific issues and see what benefits they're seeing from fasting.

fat isn't a dirty word; it's unstoppable energy!

Two words surfaced as I started researching what was happening internally during a fast: "fat-oxidation." I imagined a magical vacuum that sucks all that fat into a big, black abyss, never to be seen again. That isn't exactly what happens, but the science is just as cool and maybe a little magical. Fat oxidation is the theoretical makeover for your "extra energy," better known as fat cells, those clingy pals who've overstayed their welcome. Even after you've done a "deep cleaning," they won't budge.

Your bonus fat cells are lounging around, sipping on sugary cocktails from the last ten holiday seasons and Aunt Brenda's famous eggnog, but what we want them to do is work with us for the benefit of our body, not to its detriment. So, while we desperately try to squeeze into our favorite jeans, our fat cells feed m all the excess "energy" our body can't use to function. Look into how many calories your body needs to live for your research. It's different for each person. Anything after that number your body stores away as excess energy, but we call it fat.

I'll talk about this later, but when we don't eat or exercise, our body does not go after our stored body fat for energy. Our body's first choice is anything in the form of glucose. Its second choice is lean muscle mass. If you only exercise for 30 minutes, your body never touches your stored body fat. It uses glucose as a quick burst of energy. I won't have a chance to cover it in this book, but this is why steady-state walking is so beneficial. It never increases your heart rate, which bio-hacks your body into going to your stored body fat first. *(Look for info about the Power Five Method, where I explain everything.)* Fat oxidation is here to save the day.

ACCORDING to Dr. Dana Joffe in "The Science of Fasting," magic happens around hour twelve of a fast when the body is forced to go from sugar to fat. Joffe writes:

> "The fast-related transition, from sugar-based energy production to fat-based energy production, affects many processes in the body. For example, researchers from the Massachusetts Institute of Technology (MIT) studying mice discovered that the breakdown of fatty acids during a fast leads to the creation of new stem cells in the intestines, which help the mice recover from inflammations. Studies have also shown that processes that take place during fasting benefit pre-diabetic people, specifically by decreasing cellular insulin resistance. Ongoing studies are examining whether fasting benefits the bacterial population in our gut (the microbiome), the

development of inflammatory processes,
and maybe even to synchronize the biological clock."

ANOTHER WAY TO say that would be to picture your
body deciding it's had enough of the fluff and aches and pains
the excess fat is causing your joints. You choose to convert
those stubborn fat molecules into pure energy. It's like a
Cinderella story for your curves, turning those pumpkin-like
fat cells into the belle of the ball! Your body gets so thrilled
with the newfound energy that it starts raiding its fat stash
like a shopaholic on Black Friday. So, next time you're
fasting and begin to feel sluggish, remember that fat oxidation is your body's way of saying," Thanks for the nog, Aunt
Brenda, but you gots to go!"

Fat oxidation is a fundamental process in our bodies when
we need energy. It's like a superhero power that helps us burn
stored fat for fuel. In straightforward terms, it's the process of
breaking down fat molecules to release energy that keeps us
going.

THE FAT STORAGE: Our bodies are brilliant. They store
extra energy in the form of fat when needed, like running,
playing, or just going about their day. Think of fat as tiny
energy packets tucked away for a rainy day.

THE POWERHOUSE: *Mitochondria*: Inside our cells are
unique powerhouses called mitochondria. They're like little

factories that turn fat into energy. When your body wants to burn fat, it sends fat molecules to these factories.

THE FAT-BURNING EQUATION: Fat oxidation needs two things: oxygen and fat. Oxygen is like the key to the fat factory. When you breathe, you take in oxygen, which gets transported to the cells. Think of it as a delivery service for oxygen. Don't let me lose you in the science; let's explain the process.

- Step one: Your body signals that it needs energy, like when you start running. It sends a message to your fat cells: "We need some energy here!"
- Step two: The fat cells open up and release fat molecules into the bloodstream, like coins dropping into a vending machine.
- Step three: Oxygen from your breath and bloodstream meets these fat molecules in your cells.
- Step four: The mitochondria, those little powerhouses, work their magic and turn the fat into energy. This energy powers your muscles, heart, and all your activities.

Now that we've gotten the science part covered let's talk about the good stuff: the benefits:

Weight Loss: When you burn fat, you lose weight. It's like using up your savings.

Endurance: Fat is a long-lasting source of energy. It helps you keep going during long activities like hiking or cycling.

Balanced Energy: Fat oxidation helps stabilize your blood sugar levels, keeping you from feeling too hungry or tired.

Fat oxidation is the superhero power that helps our bodies tap into stored fat for energy. It's like breaking open piggy banks and turning fat into fuel with the help of oxygen and little powerhouses called mitochondria. So, keep moving, breathe deeply, and let your body work its fat-burning magic!

autophagy:the maintenance queen.

We will break down this "scientific" definition, and I'm going here because once we clean up the unwanted fat and break through some emotional barriers related to food, you will come back to me and ask about "maintaining results." Sister friend, "autophagy" is how we do that and much more.

Picture your ninth-grade science teacher telling you, "Autophagy is a cellular process where cells recycle their damaged components." Or if you were homeschooled, like me, you can picture your mom saying it.

If your southern, adopted Aunt Bee was telling you about it, though, she'd hand you a cup of sweet tea, invite you to the front porch swing, and say it like this:

"Well, honey, think of autophagy as a cell's way of doin' some spring cleaning. Instead of sweepin' dust under the rug or tossin' out last season's worn-out boots, cells get real smart about it. They take their broken bits and pieces and give them a good ol' recycle. Kinda like when Aunt Mabel turns her old dresses into patchwork quilts – makin' the old new again!" And we all said, "Thanks, Aunt Bee!"

Right now, weight loss is the driving force leading you to look at fasting. I'm including this short stent with another scientific term because I want you to think past your weight loss goal. Imagine you are already there: the dress/ shirt / favorite romper fits; you went to your ex's beach wedding, stunned the crowd, and no one looked at the bride. Ok, are you there? Now, look past that. What do you see? Where is your sleep, your energy, your emotional regulation?

I KNOW your bag of Skittles from the vending machine is almost empty, so suck on the last few instead of chewing them because I have two more resources I've got to share with you. This is where I will encourage you to do some research for yourself. I am not an expert on this topic, and as a whole, we are only starting to scratch the surface to understand the full benefits of fasting and auto-Nagy.

You'll want to head to whatever social platform you like to research and look up "Barbara O'Neill fasting." She has an entire multiple-part series on fasting and is considered an expert in holistic medicine.

Also read "Fast Like A Girl" by Dr. Mindy Pelz. Both women look at fasting from the weight loss perspective, but as you listen, you ask us to go further with them to look at how this will heal the body. We are starting with the idea of a one-day-a-week, 8-hour fast. These astonishing women will make a case for 18 hours and beyond fasting if you dig deeper. Understanding the science has supported my belief that this is an answer for my long-term health while also giving me the immediate results I want.

HOUR BY HOUR

When you begin an extended fast, every part of your body participates and benefits. When I found language to help me understand what was happening internally hour by hour, it helped exponentially. I included a straightforward breakdown to understand the incredible things your body is doing while taking a break from digesting. Every person is different, though, so depending on the individual, how you eat, and any other internal nuances, there will be variation.

Hour 0-12:

0-4 hours: You're still digesting your last meal. Your body is using glucose from that meal for energy.

4-12 hours: Your body starts depleting glucose stores and using glycogen (stored glucose) from your liver and muscles for energy.

Hour 12-24:

12-16 hours: Glycogen stores are running low. Your body begins to shift to burning fat for energy.

16-24 hours: The transition to burning fat continues. Ketones, a byproduct of fat metabolism, start to be produced.

Hour 24-48:

24-36 hours: Ketone levels rise. Your brain and muscles begin to use ketones more efficiently for energy. Insulin levels drop, promoting fat breakdown.

36-48 hours: Ketosis deepens. Your body increasingly relies on fat and ketones. Autophagy, a process where cells clean out damaged components, ramps up.

Hour 48-72:

48-60 hours: Ketone production is at its peak. Your body is fully adapted to burning fat for energy, and autophagy continues at a high level.

60-72 hours: Insulin levels remain low. Growth hormone levels increase, aiding in fat metabolism and muscle preservation. The body becomes very efficient at using ketones for energy.

After 72 hours, your body is in deep ketosis and significant autophagy, with high growth hormone levels to help maintain muscle mass. Refeeding after such a fast should be done gradually to avoid digestive issues.

Did you know your body could do all of that? Studying

and seeing the benefits of fasting has solidified my belief that there is a solution to any problem we face. We need to be willing to find it.

you can't use methods from 1984 and expect to get results in 2024. It's time for an upgrade!

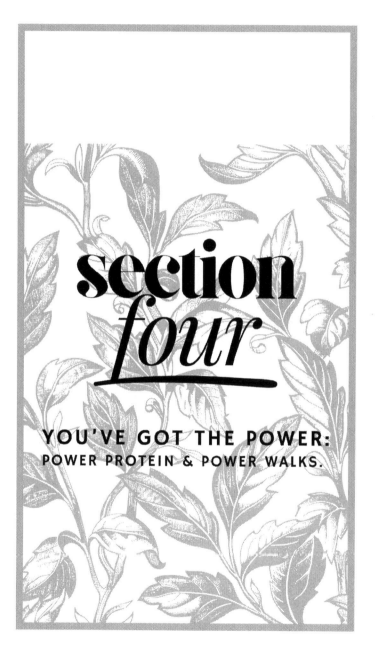

section *four*

YOU'VE GOT THE POWER:
POWER PROTEIN & POWER WALKS.

seven

. . .

Power Protein

You are about to learn how to harness the power of protein to get incredible results. It is no secret that food, exercise, and water are crucial elements of any health plan. The parts cloaked in mystery are 'What do I eat?', 'What kind of exercise?', and 'How much water do I drink?'

In "Power: walk, water, protein," we are hitting the 'delete' button on confusion and focusing on the basics you're already doing daily so you can see extraordinary results.

When we eliminate marketing confusion and colliding opinions from ego-driven trainers or nutritionists, you find the most straightforward formula for success. One of the most liberating aspects of my health journey has been connecting with experts who keep food, nutrition, and results very simple.

The Fasted Way Method's principles are as follows: You have to eat - we're simply going to eat protein. Does that feel like an oversimplification? In a way, it is, but simultaneously, it isn't. However, I promise this will make your life "simpler," while I cannot promise that creating this new habit will be easy. You're making one switch: prioritize protein first. Second, you have to exercise. I will show you how steady-state walking supersedes almost any other form of movement in the beginning stages of weight loss.]

You've heard this before: 'Eat more protein. ' Most of us understand the role of this macronutrient and why it's important. But have you had a moment where the 'theory' becomes real life, and you see the effect on the scale? I've had two of these moments and want to share them with you.

One of the last things to go before I started seeing weight loss results was the the 80/20 rule. There are so many things I love about selling supplements, but it was something I learned to say to customers because I didn't know what else to tell them besides "Take the supplements."It was more of an excuse not to pay attention to what I eat.

After working with my strength coach for six months, I hadn't seen the decrease on the scale I thought I would, and my "mom-pooch" was still pooching. So, I asked her about exercises to flatten my stomach.

I hated her answer: "Abs are made in the kitchen." I can confirm that the combination of fasting and protein has drastically decreased the mom pooch, but more importantly, the uncomfortable bloating that seems to come with constantly eating my kids' leftovers.

HOW PROTEIN WORKS IN THE BODY:

Protein is an essential macronutrient in building and repairing tissues, producing enzymes and hormones, and supporting overall body functions. When you consume protein, your body breaks it down into amino acids, which are then used to repair muscles and other tissues. This process is vital for maintaining muscle mass, especially when trying to lose weight.

HOW PROTEIN SUPPORTS MUSCLE

Muscle is metabolically active, meaning it burns calories even at rest. By supporting muscle growth and repair, protein helps boost your metabolism, making it easier to lose weight and keep it off. Additionally, maintaining muscle mass can prevent the decrease in metabolic rate that often accompanies weight loss.

BY SURRENDERING

I gave in, tired of working hard and not seeing the payoff. The first place she started was focusing on protein intake daily. I began to see the scale decrease. My family and I had a big month of travel a few months later. Traveling automatically puts routines and nutrition out of whack, and most will gain at least five pounds.

I was determined not to participate in that trend. I'd worked too hard for every pound lost. We had a Cabo vacation, a road trip to see college friends, and a 260-hour road trip with a 10-day stop to visit family.

I ended up LOSING THREE POUNDS. It solidified that even the craziest scenarios that should knock you off course can be supported by prioritizing protein.

WHEN LIFE THROWS You Curve Balls: SWING!

Most people spend a lot of time transporting. Life on the go can make sticking to a routine and nutrition difficult. Let's cover a few ways to still get in our daily protein while on the go. You'll want to plan your food for life in the car beforehand. Get protein-friendly snacks that have a minimum of 20 gr per serving. Protein bars and premade shakes are quick grabs that require nothing of you. Also, it is preferable if your food only requires one hand since one should be on the wheel. I know you think that's unnecessary to write, but how will you explain "knee driving" when you get pulled over because you were eating a salad with a fork while driving? It was a yogurt cup, and yes, I got a ticket. Please don't make my mistake; grab a protein shake.

Ready-made protein drinks, a large protein powder canister, and a trusty shaker bottle are a must, whether you are on a road trip to see family or your day is unpredictable with drop-offs and errands. Going on a family trip to visit friends or relatives out of town can be tricky if you aren't in your kitchen. It can be hard to ensure you get all the daily protein in. When it was time for my 'protein,' that protein powder saved me.

From this moment forward, there are no "cheat days." Strike the phrase "cheat meal" or "cheat day" from your vocabulary. By now, you've seen that this method is not about deprivation. It is about prioritization. Our bodies can only handle so many calories. Any excess not used for fuel or burned off by activity is stored as fat.

If you travel for work, prioritize meals if you know there will be 'dinners out' or special family days with favorite family recipes. You'll plan to get your protein early in the day, keep it simple on anything not made from the Earth, and when you sit down to a pasta feast at your boss's favorite restaurant, you know you've set yourself up for success.

There is no 'cheating' science. Your body needs what your body needs. However, we cannot ignore food's social and emotional impact. A life without fun food, social gatherings, and food freedom is a miserable way to live life.

Food is fuel, but it's also fun. When we fuel correctly 90% of the time, holidays, vacations, or nights out with friends don't derail us.

5 BENEFITS OF PROTEIN FOR WEIGHT LOSS.

1. Preserve Lean Muscle Mass: Protein is your muscle's best friend! While shedding fat helps ensure you're not losing that hard-earned muscle. Think of it as a bodyguard, ensuring your strength stays intact while the fat takes a hike.

2. Boosts Metabolism: Eating protein can help you burn more calories by digesting it. It's like your metabolism getting a mini workout every time you eat—without even hitting the gym!

3. Keeps You Feeling Full: Protein is super satisfying, so it can help you avoid those sneaky snack attacks. It's like giving your hunger a "thanks, but no thanks" response when it tries to crash your progress.

4. Supports Fat Loss, Not Muscle Loss: By prioritizing protein, you send a clear message to your body: "We're losing fat, not muscle!" This helps you stay strong and toned while the extra fat gradually disappears.

5. Stabilizes Energy Levels: Protein helps maintain steady blood sugar levels, so there are no more energy rollercoasters! You'll feel more balanced and ready to face the day without needing that third cup of coffee... unless you like coffee.

Enjoy your protein-packed meals, knowing they're working hard to support your goals—one delicious bite at a time!

. . .

THE ONE-GRAM RULE

You will start with one hundred grams of protein daily for The Fasted Way Method, but you won't stop there. Gradually, you will increase protein to one gram per pound of desired body weight. This may drive some macro enthusiasts crazy that we aren't discussing balancing carbs and fats simultaneously. However, this book isn't for them; it's for you, and you are pressed for time in your everyday life. For now, grab the "Fast On Track" Progress Tracker because it outlines how to ensure you get your protein.

For some of you, the idea of prioritizing protein is new. Depending on your age, it may be your first time hearing it. It wasn't until the rise of bodybuilding in the 1980s that sports science started to filter into mainstream living. In 1990, the general public adopted strength training, and with it, the discovery of taking more protein. The 2000s thought, with the rise of CrossFit and functional movement, brought protein into focus for people like you and me. You probably didn't realize that we have been experiencing the phenomenon of sports science infiltrating how regular people live every day.

BUT I'M NOT ARNOLD!!!

"I'll be back!" The emphasis line from The Terminator movies and Arnold Schwarzenegger's bodybuilding physique convinced aerobic-obsessed women everywhere that protein would make you look like Arnold. In 2024, I can hear the electric blue spandex you wore for your Richard Simmons workouts threatening "I'll be back," while you choose to adopt science as the foundation for your weight loss plan instead of trends led by celebrities.

Suppose we go back to the idea of "calories to live"; it's up to you how to divide those calories. I learned from several nutritionists that prioritizing protein can lessen the focus on how many carbs you eat. I incorporated that thought into The Fasted Way Method to test it out. I am so happy to tell you the theory is spot on. It has worked for me and every woman I've been able to coach through this method. Not one of the women I've helped has put a focus on 1. Counting calories, or 2. I was worrying about consuming carbs. None of them are lifting weights. Except for a few, all have lost ten pounds or more within their first forty-five days. None of them look like Arnold, I can assure you!

The reason prioritizing protein works in this way is so simple. You need food to live. When you choose food with a higher nutritional benefit, your body responds precisely how you want it to. Because protein is more filling, and your body has to work harder to break it down, your appetite is satisfied when you eat enough of it and reach for the typical, over-consumption foods less.

It's all about being intentional with your choices regarding getting the most out of your protein intake. Not all protein sources are created equal, and your choice can significantly affect how you feel and perform. The goal isn't just to eat more protein—it's to choose the right kinds that support your health and fitness goals and keep you satisfied throughout the day. From lean meats to nutrient-packed plant-based options, building various protein sources into your meals is critical to staying on track and enjoying what you eat.

For those looking to keep things simple, lean meats like chicken, turkey, and beef are excellent options for meeting your protein needs. Fish like salmon, tuna, and cod not only deliver high-quality protein but also offer a healthy dose of omega-3s, which are fantastic for overall well-being. Eggs,

Greek yogurt, and cottage cheese are easy-to-find, versatile options that add protein to any meal. Plant-based options like lentils, tofu, tempeh, and quinoa are also nutrient power-houses, making them ideal for diversifying their diet while still hitting protein targets.

And let's not forget about the benefits of fatty proteins like salmon, grass-fed beef, and whole eggs. These foods bring much more than just protein—they're packed with essential fats that support brain function, reduce inflammation, and improve overall heart health. Plus, they're full of important vitamins like A, D, and E, helping you feel nourished from the inside out. So when you add these protein-rich foods to your meals, you're not just fueling your body—you're giving it a range of nutrients that keep you energized and strong.

Incorporating a balanced variety of protein sources fuels your body for long-term health and daily performance. Whether you're grilling a piece of chicken, cooking up a salmon fillet, or tossing some tofu into a stir-fry, you're making choices that support your goals while keeping your meals flavorful and enjoyable. Protein isn't just about hitting numbers—it's about nourishing yourself with foods you love, helping you stay strong and satisfied every step of the way. For some of my favorite easy protein meal preps, go to www.thefastedway.com.

eight

. . .

Walk Don't Run

I remember the relief I felt as I listened to multiple strength coaches share the benefits of walking. After pushing myself to "go hard or go home" running the half-marathon, I laughed at something so simple that I'd made it so complicated.

IN YOUR FIRST 120 days of employing The Fasted Way Method, we don't discuss exercise. The word 'exercise' has been replaced with 'Movement,' I want you to move your body. How much have you moved your body when you get to the end of a busy day? Remember, we are keeping the mind-body connection at the center of everything. There are days you'll need a walk for your mental health. There are days you'll need a walk because your body requires a calorie deficit to lose weight. There will be days you'll need to take a walk because consistency is critical, and if this method required you to go to the gym, you would skip, but all you have to do is put one foot in front of the other for one mile. You can do that.

. . .

WALKING IS one of the most straightforward and accessible forms of exercise, yet its health benefits are often underestimated. It requires no special equipment, gym membership, or fancy technique—just a good pair of shoes and a willingness to move. Walking regularly can profoundly impact physical and mental health, making it a cornerstone of any balanced fitness routine. Whether you aim to lose weight, improve your cardiovascular health, or clear your head, walking provides a gentle yet effective way to support your overall well-being.

ONE OF THE best aspects of walking is that it can be tailored to any fitness level. There's no need to sprint or power walk your way through a workout—steady-state walking is easier on the body and can be more sustainable over time. Unlike more intense forms of exercise, walking doesn't tax the joints or leave you gasping for breath. Instead, it offers a steady, comfortable pace that keeps your heart rate in a fat-burning zone without overwhelming your system. Steady-state walking can often be more effective for fat loss than intense power walking because it keeps your body in a zone that burns fat more efficiently without triggering stress responses like cortisol release.

THE CONCEPT of "getting in your steps" took off with the advent of fitness trackers and the famous goal of reaching 10,000 steps daily. The idea can be traced back to a Japanese marketing campaign in the 1960s, where a pedometer called "mango-kei," which translates to "10,000 steps meter," was introduced. The target of 10,000 steps wasn't based on scientific research at the time but was more of a catchy goal to encourage movement. Over time, however, research has shown that this step goal correlates with significant health benefits, including improved cardiovascular health, better mood, and even a reduced risk of chronic diseases.

ONE OF THE reasons walking is so effective for weight loss is its role in creating a calorie deficit. When you walk, your body burns calories, and if you're consistently burning more than you're consuming, you'll lose weight. What's particularly great about walking is that it's a low-impact activity that you can easily incorporate into your daily routine without feeling like you're "working out." Whether it's a brisk morning walk, walking during lunch, or a relaxed evening stroll, these steps add up and contribute to your overall energy expenditure. This gradual and consistent calorie burn helps you sustainably manage your weight—without the exhaustion of intense exercise.

BEYOND THE APPARENT benefits of calorie burning, walking uniquely relates to metabolism. It helps keep the lining of your metabolism healthy and functioning optimally. Walking encourages blood flow and improves insulin sensitivity, so your body is better at processing glucose and converting it into energy rather than storing it as fat. This, in turn, helps regulate your metabolism and can even prevent metabolic diseases like type 2 diabetes. In other words, walking is like giving your metabolism a daily tune-up.

. . .

UNLIKE HIGH-INTENSITY WORKOUTS, which can sometimes leave you feeling depleted, walking leaves you energized and refreshed. It's an activity that complements your body's natural rhythms rather than working against them. Powerful or intense walking can sometimes shift your body into stress mode, raising cortisol levels, which might interfere with fat loss efforts. Steady-state walking, however, keeps stress levels low and allows you to maintain consistent, low-intensity movement for extended periods, which is critical for long-term fat-burning and health benefits.

MENTALLY, walking is a powerful tool for managing stress and boosting mood. It lets you clear your mind, reflect, or enjoy the outdoors. Many people find that walking helps alleviate anxiety, improves focus, and boosts creativity. It's a way to reset mentally while still being physically active, and there's no pressure to "perform" in the way that some high-intensity workouts demand. With walking, you set the pace, literally and figuratively, allowing for a more mindful, stress-free experience.

WALKING ALSO PLAYS a vital role in maintaining joint health. Unlike running or other high-impact activities, walking is gentle on the knees, hips, and ankles. It is an excellent option for people with joint pain or seeking a lower-impact exercise routine. Walking helps keep your joints lubricated and can even reduce the risk of arthritis as it strengthens the muscles around the joints, providing them with more support.

· · ·

FROM A CARDIOVASCULAR PERSPECTIVE, walking strengthens your heart and lungs. Even though it's low-impact, walking can still increase your heart rate enough to improve circulation and boost cardiovascular fitness. Regular walking has been shown to lower blood pressure, improve cholesterol levels, and reduce the risk of heart disease. Every step you take is a small investment in a healthier heart.

ONE OF THE best things about walking is its accessibility. You can walk almost anywhere—around your neighborhood, in a park, or at the grocery store. There's no need for special equipment, and you can do it alone or with friends, making it a highly flexible form of exercise. You don't have to carve out an hour at the gym; you can incorporate walking into your daily routine by parking farther away, taking the stairs, or going for a short walk after meals. It's all about finding small opportunities to move throughout your day.

IN ADDITION to the physical benefits, walking helps support mental clarity and emotional well-being. Studies have shown that walking can reduce symptoms of depression and anxiety, mainly due to the release of endorphins and the meditative nature of the activity. The rhythm of your steps, the fresh air, and the simple act of moving forward can create a sense of calm and help you process thoughts more effectively. Whether you're dealing with a busy mind or need a break from the stresses of daily life, walking offers a quiet space for mental restoration.

· · ·

FINALLY, one of the lesser-known benefits of walking is improving digestion. A light walk after a meal can aid digestion by stimulating your digestive system and helping food move through your stomach more efficiently. This not only prevents uncomfortable bloating but also promotes better nutrient absorption. So, next time you feel sluggish after a meal, consider taking a walk instead of sitting down—your stomach will thank you!

"Every step you walk above 4,000 per day reduces your risk of dying early by 15%," says Dr. James DiNicolantonio, author of the book 'The Obesity Fix.'

"Walking between 6,000 and 13,000 steps per day cuts the risk of dying early in half!"

INCORPORATING regular walking into your routine is a powerful, gentle way to support your overall health. It's an exercise that meets you where you are, allowing you to move at your own pace while reaping significant benefits. Walking offers a sustainable and enjoyable way to stay active, whether focused on weight loss, cardiovascular health, or healthy metabolism. Plus, you get to enjoy the journey with each step you take!

nine

. . .

Wonder Working Water

Y ou've said it, I've said it, and I've heard it said to me hundreds of times, "But when I drink water, I need to pee all the time." Maybe we are collectively holding onto PTSD from constantly going to the bathroom during pregnancy. Perhaps we don't want to be inconvenienced.

What I hope to highlight for you with this last pillar of The Fasted Way Method are some ideas that will encourage you to push past the inevitable treks to the bathroom and the inconvenience. You may want to buy a designated cup with bright colors to be visually reminded to grab and drink it when you see it. I can tell you that not drinking water will, at worst, sabotage your best weight loss efforts and, at best, will slow your results.

———

WATER IS OFTEN HAILED as the unsung hero in the battle for better health, and when it comes to weight loss, it's more important than ever. Water is crucial in helping your body process and move fat out of the body, primarily by supporting the liver and kidneys—two organs critical for metabolizing fat. When you're well-hydrated, your liver can convert stored fat into energy more effectively, and your kidneys efficiently filter waste. Without enough water, your body struggles to break down fat, making it harder to lose weight. So yes, water helps you flush fat away—maybe not as quickly as we'd all like!

BUT EXACTLY HOW much water should you be drinking? The general recommendation is around **8 cups (64 ounces) per day**, though your specific needs can vary based on weight, activity level, and climate. Some experts suggest aiming for **half your body weight in ounces** of water. So, if you weigh 150 pounds, that's about 75 ounces daily. And if you're sweating it out during workouts or living in a hot climate, you'll need even more to stay hydrated.

IF YOU'RE A COFFEE LOVER, here's a pro tip: for every cup of coffee, you'll want to drink an extra glass of water. Coffee, while glorious for waking us up in the morning, is a diuretic, meaning it can lead to dehydration by making you lose more water. Balancing your coffee intake with extra water helps counteract that dehydrating effect. Think of it as the water doing damage control for your caffeine fix!

NOW, let's talk about hydration's archenemies—the sneaky things that can dry you out and sabotage your efforts. First on the list **sugar**. Sugary drinks, sodas, and processed snacks provide empty calories and pull water from your body as it metabolizes. **Alcohol** is another well-known dehydrator, as anyone who's woken up parched after a night out can attest. **High-sodium foods** (think processed and packaged meals) are also culprits, as they cause your body to retain water, leading to that bloated feeling while still leaving you dehydrated. Lastly, don't forget about **vigorous exercise** without proper rehydration. Sweating out water without replenishing it can quickly tip the scales toward dehydration.

ONE TRICK for staying hydrated and boosting your mineral intake is adding a pinch of **pink Himalayan salt** to your water. Unlike regular table salt, which is heavily processed, Himalayan salt contains over 80 trace minerals, including magnesium, calcium, and potassium, which help regulate hydration and balance electrolytes. These minerals are essential if you're sweating a lot, as they deplete through perspiration. Adding just a tiny pinch to your water can help your body absorb and retain the water you drink more efficiently.

SALT ALSO PLAYS a crucial role in balancing pH levels in the body. Alkalizing your system helps reduce inflammation and supports healthy digestion. If you struggle to drink enough water because it just doesn't taste interesting, a little salt can also give your water a slight but refreshing flavor boost, making it easier to sip throughout the day.

. . .

IT'S essential to remember that dehydration can sneak up on you, and even mild dehydration can have surprising effects on your body. From sluggish metabolism to poor digestion and even increased hunger, being dehydrated can mimic many symptoms of hunger, leading you to eat more when your body craves water. So before you reach for that snack, try drinking a glass of water first—you might find that your hunger has disappeared.

THE BEST PART about staying hydrated? It's one of the easiest things to do to support weight loss. Drinking water helps you feel fuller, reduces your appetite, and prevents overeating. Also, when you're hydrated, your body has more energy to move, exercise, and burn calories throughout the day. Even mild dehydration can cause fatigue, so keeping your water bottle handy helps you stay energized and active.

LET'S not forget the skin benefits. Staying hydrated gives your skin a healthy, glowing look; water helps flush out toxins and keep skin cells plump. So, not only does water help you move fat out of your body, but it can also make you look fresher and more vibrant in the process. Think of water as a natural, no-cost beauty treatment!

SO WHETHER YOU'RE sipping it plain, spicing it up with a bit of pink salt, or drinking an extra glass to make up for your morning coffee, water is your best friend in your weight loss journey. Keep it flowing, and your body will thank you with better energy, clearer skin, and even that little extra boost toward your fat loss goals!

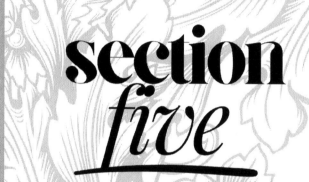

section five

THE FASTED WAY IN ACTION

ten

. . .

Let's Map It!

E mbarking on a 120-day fasting schedule can be a powerful way to reshape your habits and jumpstart sustainable weight loss. Committing to one 8-hour fast per week and walking at least 1 mile sets the stage for gradual, steady progress.

Research shows it takes about 66 to 120 days to form and solidify new habits, so this schedule gives your body and mind the time needed to adjust and thrive. During this period, you can expect meaningful changes, not just in the number on the scale but also in how you feel—more energized, focused, and in control of your health. Although results vary, this combination of fasting and light activity can lead to consistent weight loss as your body adapts to using fat stores for energy during fasts.

At the same time, walking helps boost your metabolism and overall calorie burn. This approach is gentle yet effective, making it a sustainable strategy for long-term health improvement.

your first 30 days are for adjusting

Can you lose weight during this time? Yes, but that isn't the goal. Your primary focus will be adjusting and consistently doing the daily activities. One of my favorite things about this method is that it doesn't require perfection from you to see results. You will quickly see where your gaps are and what you may need to adjust in your daily life to get your walking in or drink all your water.

SET *yourself up for success by starting your first thirty days to adjust to something new.*

your 30-day plan

- 1. One 8-HR fast per week.
- 2. Drink 90 oz of water.
- 3. Eat 100 grams of protein per day.
- 4. Walk 1 mile every day.

Some of you will read that list and feel relieved; others will think it's too simple. This is a crucial rule: Don't do it if you cannot sustain something during a life-curve ball moment. This week, you may be able to handle walking further or fasting longer. However, if sickness hits your house next week, are you more likely to get in a 1-mile or 3-mile walk? Returning to Set Point Theory, you want to be gentle with your approach as you start incorporating new routines.

. . .

IF YOU ARE USUALLY VERY active, you can walk 3,000 steps daily, roughly 2 miles, and about 40 minutes of steady-state walking.

THESE FIRST THIRTY days will highlight how you deal with stress more than you do anything. Starting these four steps is not for stress relief. In "Just Don't," several ways are listed to deal with stress in non-eating and non-spending ways. Yes, walking can be a great way to deal with stress, but you'll want to slow down and have a few tools in your belt that you can employ quickly.

DAYS 31-60
1. One 24-HR fast and three 8-HR fasts.
2. 90 oz of water.
3. 100 grams of protein.
4. Walk 2 miles every day.

YOUR 24-HOUR *fast will look something like this:*

SUNDAY EVENING: Eat dinner.
Monday morning: Drink water.
Monday night: bed-time at 9:00 PM
Tuesday morning: Break your fast with fatty protein, carbs like fruit, and good fats. That will count towards your 100 grams of protein for the day. For the rest of the day, you'll want to make sure you eat the rest of your 100 grams. Don't be afraid to eat other food. Just eat normally and stick with prioritizing protein.

. . .

DAYS 61-90
1. One 48-HR fast and three 8-HR fasts.
2. 90 oz of water.
3. 100 grams of protein.
4. Walk 3 miles per day.

DAYS 91-120
1. One 72-HR fast and three 8-HR fasts.
2. 90 oz of water.
3. 100 grams of protein.
4. Walk 4 miles per day.

troubleshoot

My first attempt at an 8-HR fast ended at 3:00 PM, and I found myself binging Hawaiian Rolls in the pantry. My first attempt at a 72-hour fast ended after 48 hours. It is so important to know when to call it quits. Yes, you will want to complete the fasts you set out to do, but I have only accomplished a 40-pound weight loss because of how many fasts I've failed.

YOU ARE GOING to learn so much about yourself. The only way you lose is if you don't see yourself through and keep trying. Over the summer, my goal was to finish losing the last ten pounds that were holding on for dear life. Simultaneously, I was figuring out how to run a small business and gathering resources to start homeschooling my daughter; my husband was in a 'busy season,' meaning I was single-parenting a lot while he fulfilled his work obligations. We were transitioning my special needs son from public to private school, and I hosted a group of moms and kids at my house every week to learn and play.

I TEND to wake up through the night when my life is complete. One of the calming techniques for me is taking a bath. I know this about myself. However, I forgot. On Day 2 of a 72-hour fast, I woke around 2 am. My priority is, 'How can I quickly get back to sleep?' This has been one of the hardest things to overcome while I'm on a fast. I ended up eating something and ending my fast short of my goal. The following month, it was time for another 72-hour fast. This time, I reminded myself before I went to sleep, "If you wake up, take a bath. If you still can't sleep, eat something." I did wake up that night, and I remembered to take a bath before heading to the pantry. I got right back in bed and completed my 72-hour fast.

HEAT HAS ALSO BEEN an enormous help. I've learned so much about my nervous system and individual needs. My body is wired for the heat. Summer is my favorite season, and 100-degree days with my kids in the pool are my happy place. As I head into the fall and winter this year, I've made some mental notes to ensure I get an excellent Vitamin D supplement and buy a heating pad.

ALL OF THOSE things fall under the category of "support!" As you take one step at a time, you will notice the things you gravitate towards that help you find calm and the things or people that trigger stress in your body. Two of the triggers I found out about myself in the last six months that I had to stay away from if I'm fasting because stress in my body sends hunger cues to my brain are talking about finances with my husband and political controversies on social media. The next time I was fasting, I front-loaded the conversation with my husband and asked if he could wait till I was done fasting to bring up anything about finances. I also deleted a few social media apps that I enjoy but didn't want the stress of political drama on a fast.

hunger

You could move through this 120-day fasting schedule without setbacks in an ideal world. However, you are not a robot, and life happens. It may take you six weeks to work up to your 48-hour fast or five months to reach your 72-hour fast. When creating a plan, the model is always going to be linear. Still, reality will have peaks and valleys, highs and lows, with your primary job being to live somewhere in the middle by prioritizing consistency over anything else. Enjoy the highs, but know you're going to come back down. Embrace the lows and learn what you can, but put out the 'Welcome' mat and live there.

DEPENDING ON YOUR METABOLISM, you may get hungrier faster than others on this journey. Remember that the calories your body needs are unique to you. It would be best if you weren't hungry on your non-fasting days. If you increase your protein by ten grams for that week, watch how you feel. The scale should not increase more than 1-2 pounds. If you feel satisfied with that protein amount, stay there for a few weeks and assess again. When you notice your body showing those same hunger cues, increase by ten grams of protein. You'll want to weigh to see that there aren't any spikes in weight.

YOUR GOAL IS to work up to your personal protein goal. The formula I shared above is the simplest way I can share how to do that without making crazy adjustments to your diet or needing customizing macros.

signs to watch for

If you consistently gain and lose the same five pounds as you go through this process, here are a few signs to watch for and adjustments you can make. Keep A Food Journal

Sometimes, the normal food we've been eating prevents us from seeing the results we really want. Your goal isn't to eliminate food. Your goal is to listen to your body. If you consistently gain and lose the same weight, your body is trying to tell you that it can burn everything you're consuming. You can always follow the formula for increasing protein first and see if that helps fill the hunger gap you may be filling.

walk the line

Like Johnny Cash told June, "I walk the line." Walking and fasting are your two avenues to help your body get into a calorie deficit. Ask yourself, "Am I reaching my daily walking goal?" If yes, you may increase your daily walking goal by half a mile. If those two options are not helping your body maintain the number you hit after a fast, then you can look at eliminating something for one week.

HERE ARE *a few things you could try for five days; you'll choose one:*

- Eliminate dairy
- Eliminate processed sugar.
- Eliminate soda.
- Eliminate fast food/eating out.
- Eliminate alcohol.
- Eliminate processed carbs (breads and pasta.)

IF YOU NEED A 5-DAY ELIMINATION, ensure you have an abundance of fruits, veggies, and ready-to-go protein. Hunger is excellent because it lets you know your metabolism works, but you should only be ravenously hungry sometimes.

the most important tip i have to give you

As I've coached women, I've seen this tendency to want to do more or add to a desire to see results faster. My biggest tip would be to follow the 120-day fasting schedule with as much consistency as possible without adding additional exercise or nutrition plans. When we bounce from one thing to another, we put our minds in constant problem-solving, which is the opposite of rest. You may see how much you don't rest on this journey. You may uncover that being still is hard for you and that you need busyness and a constantly full schedule to feel productive. I can tell you we are not designed to be in a never-ending sprint mode. We are designed for rest, especially rest in our minds.

the final tortilla

We are wrapping this up!

You were made for this moment, friend. Your physical body is something to be nurtured, cherished, and loved. If you hate your body, it will translate to your decisions. Switching our minds from forcing our bodies to perform with extreme methods to meeting our bodies' needs may be the most excellent flex of your lifetime.

YOU ARE MAKING A DIFFERENCE. The next time you are at dinner with your girlfriends, you will probably hear all the different ideas about weight loss, trends, and what someone has seen on social media. In that moment, know that you are choosing something different for yourself. Change is difficult, but you are the right woman for the job. Your body is not broken; it needs the right tools to succeed. I know you are committed to getting those tools.

i believe in you!

section
six

11 SECRETS TO KNOW
WHEN FASTING FOR WEIGHT LOSS

eleven

. . .

The Beta Group

Before social platforms, "going viral" meant you were ill, and the Grim Reaper was probably on his way to ring your doorbell. The modern interpretation of the term has taken on a whole new meaning, though. I've been on social media for over twenty years when you had to have a college email to even have a social media account, and "Myspace" was the original blog. Posting my life and thoughts has been a regular part of my adult life. However, the "viral" social media waterfall was unknown until I shared a picture of my results using what you now know as 'The Fasted Way Method.'

IN AUGUST OF 2023, I shared my shock over my results with fasting. The post was flooded with comments, and I couldn't keep up with the messages. I thought, 'What if I could help some of these women get the same results I've gotten with fasting.' I didn't have anything written down. There weren't any ebooks or video courses. I coached each of them one-on-one on customizing their plan and personally troubleshot with them weekly to help them maximize their results. I'm still shocked by their results.

In her late forties, Cheri lost seven pounds in a weekend and maintained that through three weeks of travel. She then accomplished her first three-day fast and shared, "I never thought I would've been able to do this without your support and this method."

Stacey, a thirty-nine-year-old mother and small business owner, lost seventeen pounds in her first thirty days. That one floored me. She had been so frustrated with where her body ended up after having kids late in life that she shared she was overjoyed to find something she could do in her busy life. As of November 2023, Stacey had lost twenty-two pounds.

Liberty, a twenty-something professional, was tired of trying all the programs but not seeing success. She lost seven pounds in her first week. When life started to get complicated with the loss of a loved one and the business of work, she said everything was easy to maintain. She continued to see success.

It was one thing to see success with the knowledge I'd gained working with experts. Being able to help others see the same success has resulted in an accidental business and a system made up of physical books, journals, study guides, and online video courses. You would not be reading this book without that initial group of women who were willing to trust me and take a bit of a wild ride.

twelve

. . .

eleven secrets to know when you're fasting for
weight loss

As you work through fasting, you will find tips and tricks to add to your list of 'how to's". There are a few that I would add to this list that are specific to me, like 'be ok with your kids eating chicken nuggets from the air fryer' instead of anything that requires you to stand over the stove and smell food. We would catalog that under the 'cruel and unusual punishment' category. This list is also objective. As is true of this method, there are cold hard truths that will not change, and then there are interpretations that will make your journey unique to you. Use these eleven tips as a foundation to jump-start your list. Keep what works for you, discard what doesn't, and add your own.

secret one : prepare to fail and be disappointed

You may be a mythical unicorn who does everything well the first time. For the rest of us mortals, anything new we do takes time to explore how we will respond. Like going into labor with your first child, you can think you know, but everything has only been a theory until you're feeling that first contraction. I "failed" my first fasting day in June 2023 and then binge-ated everything in my pantry. However, I had to have my "first day". The next time, I was successful because I knew what to expect, and the results were undeniable.

secret two: black coffee is your best friend.

But if you need creamer, that's okay. I have had an insane sugar addiction for the majority of my life. It's rooted in stress. When I started fasting, I drank coffee but had to have creamer. When I wanted to see results in September, I gave up the creamer and started drinking it black. I wouldn't say I liked it. However, the benefits were worth the sacrifice. The black coffee gave me an energy boost and suppressed my appetite. Ten months later, I haven't returned to creamer in my coffee.

secret three: tell somebody.

If you live with another human, let them know your fasting days. If you're a mom, you may want to ask your husband to be in charge of dinner and stay out of the kitchen. If you have a roommate who likes to grab you something sweet from your local spot, tell them you must put a clothespin on your nose and take a cold shower if they walk in with donuts. My husband and I love late-night ice cream after the kids go to bed. If I see him grab his keys and head towards the front door at 8:30 PM, I must tell him, "Don't get my any." This will be a great place to start if you aren't used to communicating your needs.

secret four: embrace grace, not willpower.

You have done plenty of programs that you have had to force yourself to do the uncomfortable. It would be best if you didn't do that with fasting. We are not gentle or kind with our bodies. Fasting is one of the kindest things you could do for your body because it allows your digestive system to rest and cells to heal. Start the day permitting yourself to listen and explore your limitations. Then, decide if you need to stop or have enough mental capacity to step beyond that barrier into a new place. Ultimately, this is up to you. No one is telling you that shattering your comfort zone is the way to achieve success here.

secret five: drink water... no, i'm serious!

Yes, you will have to pee a lot. BUT THAT IS HOW FAT LEAVES YOUR BODY. When we drink plenty of water while fasting, our bodies go after our stored body fat for energy. When we consume enough water for all our organs to function, it begins releasing broken-down fat into our blood-stream. So, as you are peeing more than you would, imagine how much fat is leaving your body. I hope you pee a lot :)

secret six: prepare to surprise yourself!

While this will be hard for most, perhaps less hard for others, the part that will bring you joy and surprise is what you are capable of. Your body is capable. It is your mind that holds you back. While this isn't the place to grit your teeth and shatter your comfort zone, you must find courage and perseverance to see yourself through whether you hit your intended goal or listen to your body and stop short of it. You will need perseverance to finish.

YOU WILL NEED perseverance to start again to believe you aren't a failure and can succeed. You may surprise yourself and be able to cook dinner for the family after a complete 48-hour fast. You may surprise yourself when you finish fasting for eight hours and realize you can have your first meal at breakfast the next day. You will surprise yourself when you step on the scale. There will be a shock when you see what your body can do when you allow it to have the right tools.

secret seven: your scale is not the villain in your story.

If you have used the scale as a weapon of mass destruction against yourself, you should forego it for now. Be willing to detach emotions to the number that pops up and blinks at you instead of attaching your worth as a human being. You are not more valuable if the number goes down, and simultaneously, you are not less valuable if the number goes up. The scale is FEEDBACK! Valuable feedback. The scale lets you know what is working and what isn't. On the day of your fast, weigh first when your feet hit the floor. Then weigh again when your fast is finished before you eat your next meal. If you broke your fast with dinner, weigh again the following day. If you go, you weigh a total of 24 hours before breakfast. This isn't just going to tell you how much you lost. It will also help you know where you are to maintain the results you got. Weigh regularly.

secret eight: digestion waste is the first to go.

There are four different types of weight loss. When the word "weight" is often used, there is an immediate connection to the word "fat" in our minds; that isn't always the case. Because of the regular American diet, most of us carry up to five pounds of weight in our digestive tract. Your first fast will allow your body to let go of all it's been holding onto. You may see your stomach less swollen or feel less bloated. Bloat is often due to inflammation in the gut. When you let the body do its job, the bloat goes. In the mini-course "The Fasted Way 101," the other three types will be covered, and I'll answer questions like "How do I know if the weight I'm losing is fat?" "How often do I need to fast to burn stubborn body fat?" Info for the class will be in your inbox soon. I know you will love the tools you'll get.

secret nine: don't be a hero, sleep when you need to.

Fasting is not about proving how strong you are. It's about embracing weakness. Sometimes, I rush with energy while fasting and having a kitchen dance party with the kids. I know that if I do that, I've used up precious energy that my body needs, and if I choose to stay up past 10:00 p.m., I will be in the pantry at 9:30 p.m.

YOU WILL FEEL weak because food is energy, and you are not giving your body its typical energy source. That doesn't mean you won't be able to live your everyday life and meet the daily demands you have. It does mean that you need to be aware of what is extra. If something isn't required of you, don't do it. Conserve your energy where you can. NAP! Often, on my fasting days, I nap when my daughter does. Embrace the weakness because the real show is happening underneath the surface, invisible to the human eye.

secret ten: if you lick the spoon, keep going.

I am notorious for licking the spoon with which I make my kid's sandwiches. Unconsciously, I have habits that I do without thinking. So do you. Fasting is going to highlight your habits, all of them. Often, we walk through life as bystanders without slowing down to take inventory of the small things we do. When cooking, have a designated plate or holder for your utensils. Also, have a towel for your hands in case you are like me and have the habit of licking the peanut butter off your thumb. And if you do accidentally lick the spoon, keep going. A little "peanut butter" isn't going to ruin your efforts.

secret eleven: your stress is best friends with your fat; let yourself rest!

There is undeniable evidence that stress in the body produces the hormone called "cortisol." I won't talk about that because you can find info everywhere now. I will give you a different piece of mental pie to chew on. Stress costs you energy. Negative emotions, like stress, withdraw from the body. Positive emotions put deposits of energy into the body. There are stressors that we cannot escape. So goes the story of life. Though I love my children, I expect them to cause me stress until I find better ways to respond to the parenting challenges

I find myself in. Changing your response in those situations will take time and the ability to self-reflect with an objective viewpoint of your person and behavior. You don't want to wait to start fasting until your Mother Theresa. Don't take on any unnecessary stress while working on your responses to the beautiful halflings sharing your space with you. When I don't say no and allow my yeses to send me into mental withdrawal, I am heading to the pantry. I will eat the entire 24-pack of Hawaiian Rolls or a pint of ice cream.

WHEN FASTING AND A SITUATION, emotion, or event comes up outside your daily routine, ask yourself, "Can this wait until tomorrow?" "Is this an emergency?" "Is giving my 'yes' to this (fill in the blank) worth sabotaging my efforts?" If the answer is "Yes!" To those questions, move forward, but don't end your fast. Have a backup snack just in case, but this is an opportunity to surprise yourself. This is your body's chance to shine and show you what it's capable of. What is on the other side of that? "Yes!" Is confidence. A confident woman is hard to stop.

freebie! find rest, and i don't mean sleep.

Sometimes, on my fasting days, it is easier if the day is complete. I'm so busy moving from one thing to the next that I don't have time to think about hunger. However, mental unrest and constantly being on my feet moving around have been the end of more fasting days than I would like to remember. Realizing that you need busyness and movement to feel productive in your day might bring some uncomfortable emotions to you. Resting is more than sleep. It is a place though. At the mention of weight loss, he wanted to know more.

He was in disbelief that he could continue to eat the food he loved, incorporate fasting and walking, and lose weight. He told me he needed to lose over one hundred pounds and that he'd researched several different methods, but nothing seemed to be working for him. At one point, he said, "But I love to eat. I don't need to change my portion sizes?" I told him the principles you've read through this book and assured him I couldn't think of why this method wouldn't work for him.

As he pulled up to the drop-off spot, I reached the door handle to move on with my day. Antonio looked back one more time and said,

"Thank you! You may have just saved my life!"

Those words were a little shocking to hear, but the sincerity was evident. Not every man knows his way around a gym, and even if he does, he may not have the time to dedicate to going or the full knowledge of how to get results.

conclusion

The Fasted Way Method is the key you have been looking for to unlock the 'forever weight loss' door. Undoubtedly, we need each piece of the puzzle our body requires to operate correctly. Weight loss is a beautiful byproduct of a life lived in full. Perfection is a myth, friend, as is balance. Imbalance is what we can count on most. As we constantly strive for perfect balance in our lives in every area, we doom ourselves to failure or chasing that elusive white rabbit down a never-ending hole.

There will always be parts of your life that demand more of you in different seasons than others. When we fall 'off balance,' we don't allow space for the path to curve unexpectedly or for a 'deer' to jaunt into our path as we swerve. Where is the balance in that moment? Perhaps the word we should adopt is 'pivot'!

You will succeed if you apply the steps laid out for your first 120 days. It would be best to consider it a guarantee that the journey will not look like you imagined. There is a high possibility it will be better.

Remember, you are the right person for this moment. You have the strength and the determination to succeed with the Fasted Way Method. Embrace this opportunity and start your journey towards a healthier, happier you.

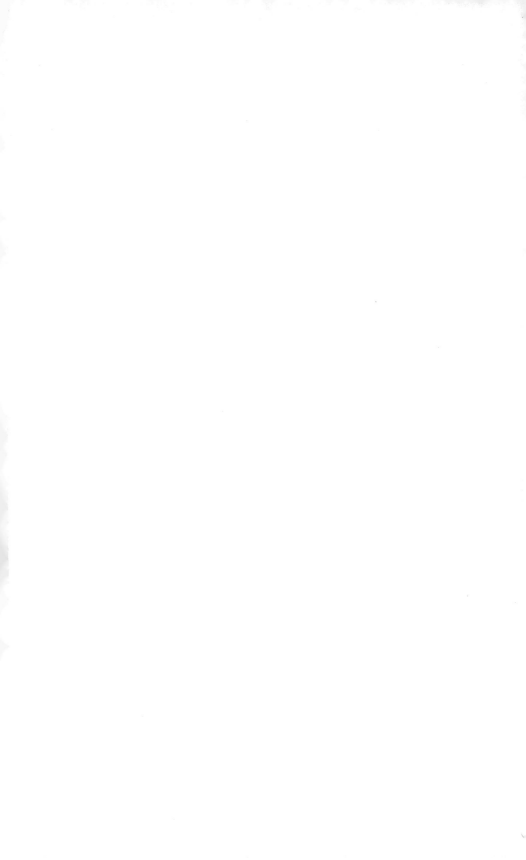

Made in the USA
Columbia, SC
30 December 2024

50878641R00080